Contents

Bovine spongiform encephalopathy

by
Richa[illegible]erlin
Scrap[illegible] Related Diseases
Advis[illegible]y Service
Edinburgh, UK

FAO ANIMAL PRODUCTION AND HEALTH PAPER

109

Food and Agriculture Organization of the United Nations

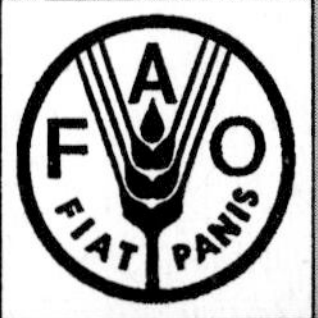

Rome, 1993

M-27
ISBN 92-5-103155-X

Acknowledgements

The author is greatly indebted to Mr John W. Wilesmith for making available a large amount of unpublished information and for supplying some of the figures; to Gerald A.H. Wells for providing original photographs; and to both gentlemen for invaluable criticism of the manuscript. The author is also grateful to the Animal Health and Veterinary Group at MAFF, Tolworth, for constructive comments and for checking the accuracy of the references to legislation.

Abbreviations

BSE
Bovine spongiform encephalopathy

CEC
Commission of the European Communities

CJD
Creutzfeldt-Jakob disease

CWD
Chronic wasting disease

DHSS
Department of Health and Social Security, UK

DoH
Department of Health, UK

EEC
European Economic Community

EM
Electron microscope

FSE
Feline spongiform encephalopathy

GSS
Gerstmann-Straussler syndrome

HMSO
Her Majesty's Stationery Office, UK

MAFF
Ministry of Agriculture, Fisheries and Food, UK

OIE
Office international des epizooties, France

SAF
Scrapie-associated fibrils

sip
Scrapie incubation period

TME
Transmissible mink encephalopathy

USDA
United States Department of Agriculture

Introduction

INTRODUCTION TO BOVINE SPONGIFORM ENCEPHALOPATHY (BSE)

BSE is a new disease of cattle. It was first recognized and defined in the United Kingdom in November 1986 by histopathological examination of affected brains (Wells *et al.*, 1987). Over the next four years, the disease developed into a large-scale epidemic in most of the country, with serious economic consequences.

BSE occurs in adult animals of both sexes, typically in four- and five-year-olds. It is a neurological disease involving pronounced changes in mental state, abnormalities of posture and movement and of sensation. The clinical disease usually lasts for several weeks and it is characteristically progressive and fatal (Wilesmith *et al.*, 1988).

The pathology of BSE immediately suggested the nature of the disease and its probable cause. Microscopic lesions in the central nervous system consist of a bilaterally symmetrical, non-inflammatory vacuolation of neuronal perikarya and grey-matter neuropil (Wells *et al.*, 1987). This is the classical picture of the scrapie family of diseases and, on this evidence alone, it seemed highly likely that BSE was a new member of the family.

BSE was subsequently shown to be experimentally transmissible to other cattle, after very long incubation periods (one to two years) by the injection of brain homogenates from clinical cases (Dawson, Wells and Parker, 1990a). This left no doubt that BSE is caused by a scrapie-like infectious agent.

Epidemiological studies showed the vehicle of infection to be meat and bone meal that had been incorporated into concentrated feedstuffs as a protein-rich supplement. The outbreak was probably started by scrapie infection of cattle, but the subsequent course of the epidemic was driven by the recycling of infected cattle material within the cattle population (Wilesmith, Ryan and Atkinson, 1991; Wilesmith and Wells, 1991).

The average level of infection to which cattle were exposed was very low. The reason why this led to such a large number of BSE cases is that much of the United Kingdom dairy cattle population was exposed for many years. There is no firm evidence for the direct transmission of infection from cattle to cattle.

In July 1988 the British Government introduced a ban on the feeding of ruminant protein to ruminants to stop the occurrence of new infections (HMSO, 1988a). However, the average incubation period of BSE is around four to five years and, as of July 1991, there had been insufficient time for the feed ban to affect the incidence of clinical disease.

Long incubation periods are a characteristic feature of all scrapie-like diseases. There is no laboratory diagnostic test for the infectious agent in live animals, mainly because of the absence of any known immune response to infection. Infected animals can only be identified when they develop the clinical disease.

The fact that BSE belongs to the scrapie family is of the greatest importance. The biochemical nature of the scrapie/BSE agent has yet to be established but many of the biological properties of these infectious agents are well understood. There are precedents among members of the scrapie family to indicate the possible future directions of the BSE epidemic and the additional measures that might be needed to eradicate it (Wilesmith and Wells, 1991).

The epidemiological relationships between the various members of the scrapie family clearly define the circumstances under which BSE might, in theory, present a risk to public health. Knowledge of the pathogenesis of these diseases shows precisely the preemptive action that can be taken to minimize this risk (Kimberlin, 1990b; 1990c).

The advent of BSE has made a sizeable impact throughout much of the world even though few countries, other than the United Kingdom, have experienced cases. Trade has been disrupted, sometimes unnecessarily, and great fears have been aroused about the possible occurrence of BSE elsewhere in the world. However a rapid increase in the understanding of the disease over the last four years leaves few unanswered questions of major practical importance. BSE can be prevented, controlled and eradicated.

TABLE 1

Spongiform encephalopathies related to BSE in chronological order of demonstrated transmissibility

Disease and occurrence	Host species	Date
Scrapie Common in several countries throughout the world	Sheep, goats	1936
Transmissible mink encephalopathy (TME) Very rare, but adult mortality nearly 100% in some outbreaks	Mink	1965
Kuru Once common among the Fore-speaking people of Papua New Guinea, now rare	Humans	1966
Creutzfeldt-Jakob disease (CJD) Uniform worldwide incidence of one per million per annum	Humans	1968
Gerstmann-Straussler syndrome (GSS) A familial form of CJD; less than 0.1 per million per annum	Humans	1981
Chronic wasting disease (CWD)* Colorado and Wyoming, USA	Mule deer, elk	1983

*Experimental transmission not demonstrated.

DISEASES RELATED TO BSE

To understand BSE requires an appreciation of some of the other diseases in the scrapie family listed in Table 1. A detailed review has recently been published (Kimberlin, 1990a). The main features of those diseases that are particularly important in the context of BSE are summarized below. Other related diseases are discussed on pages 28–30.

Scrapie

Scrapie in sheep (and goats) is the best understood member of the family. It has been endemic in the United Kingdom for over two centuries and is present in many other countries of the world.

Scrapie occurs as a natural infection of adult sheep which is transmitted maternally, from ewe to lamb. Some of this maternal transmission occurs before or at the time of parturition. But it can also occur afterwards because the incidence of scrapie in offspring increases the longer that lambs run with their ewes. Scrapie infection can also spread horizontally between unrelated sheep. With both types of transmission, the oral route of infection is one of those implicated and the placenta is one tissue known to be a source of infection. This information provides a basis for the control of scrapie using two complementary approaches.

The first control method relies on the fact that many of the lambs born to scrapie-infected ewes will themselves become infected regardless of the stage in the ewe's incubation period when they were born. With detailed breeding records, it becomes possible to cull selectively in the female line to reduce the number of sheep in the flock with a high probability of being infected.

The basis of the second approach is that a breeding ewe that is incubating scrapie will not only drop a lamb with a high risk of being infected, but an infected placenta as well. This will be a direct (through eating the placenta) and an indirect (through contamination of the lambing pasture) source of infection to other sheep that come into contact with it. The physicochemical stability of the scrapie agent means that infection can persist in the environment for a long time. Hence farmers are advised to destroy placentas as soon as possible and to keep the lambing premises clean.

Although scrapie is caused by an infectious agent, a single sheep gene (known as sip: scrapie incubation period) exerts a major influence on the length of incubation period. This gene has two alleles (sA and pA), producing three different sip genotypes of sheep. Sheep homozygous for sA are the most likely to develop the natural disease, but some heterozygotes (sApA) may succumb to the disease if the exposure to infection is high enough.

It seems highly probable that the sip gene is the same as the PrP gene which codes for the precursor of the fibril protein that forms scrapie-associated fibrils (SAF) (see Evidence for infection, p. 13 and Molecular pathology, p. 35). Biochemical markers are being developed to identify the sA and pA alleles of the sip gene with a view to the possible use of selected sires (sip pApA) as an additional approach to the control of scrapie.

The relevance of scrapie to BSE is threefold. First, scrapie is the likely origin of the BSE epidemic (see p. 22). Second, scrapie provides one of the two main scenarios for the future course of BSE and indicates the type of control measures to be considered should BSE become an endemic infection of cattle (see Control and eradication, p. 55). Third, past exposure to scrapie, which has not been a risk for human beings, provides a baseline for assessing the public health risks caused by BSE (see Creutzfeldt-Jakob disease, p. 6).

Transmissible mink encephalopathy (TME)

TME is a very rare disease of ranch-reared mink, but it can have devastating consequences, sometimes eliminating an entire herd of adult breeding animals. The disease is caused by an exogenous source of infection to which mink become exposed via contaminated feed. It is not uncommon for mink ranchers to include untreated abattoir waste and dead stock in mink feed.

Since sheep (and perhaps goats) are the only known animal reservoirs of the scrapie-like agents in nature, a direct link between scrapie and TME is likely even though it has not been possible to document the feeding of sheep material in all outbreaks. The same assumption can be made for BSE. Indeed, TME provides a precedent for the origin of BSE, although the circumstances of infection are different. The main differences are that TME is associated with rare, geographically localized, comparatively high levels of exposure to infection in untreated abattoir waste, whereas BSE (at least in the United Kingdom) is due to widespread, prolonged exposure to a very low level of infection in processed animal waste (Kimberlin, 1990b).

An important aspect of TME is that it is a "dead-end" disease with no natural routes of transmission from mink to mink, unless there is cannibalism. In this respect it differs markedly from scrapie and provides a precedent for the alternative scenario for the future course of the BSE epidemic.

Kuru

Kuru is associated with the very small population of Fore-speaking people in Papua New Guinea and it occurred in rather special circumstances. It may have originated from a spontaneous case of Creutzfeldt-Jakob disease (CJD), but the practice of ritual cannibalism of dead relatives was certainly the means by which neuropathogenic strains of the agent were "passaged" within families. An equivalent situation occurred in BSE with the recycling of infected cattle material within the cattle population. This proved to be the main factor driving the BSE epidemic (see p. 25-26).

Kuru is also important because there appear to be no other routes for the transmission of infection and the cessation of cannibalism has led to the gradual disappearance of kuru. In other words, human beings are effectively a "dead-end" host for the disease. In this respect, kuru resembles TME.

Creutzfeldt-Jakob disease (CJD)

Two other scrapie-like diseases are known in human beings, although Gerstmann-Straussler syndrome (GSS) is usually regarded as a variant of CJD (see Table 1).

CJD can occur in a familial pattern (as do GSS and scrapie) but it is typically sporadic and has a remarkably uniform incidence worldwide of about one case per million of the population per annum. The epidemiological explanation for the sporadic occurrence of CJD is uncertain but one important possibility has been eliminated.

Because of the precedent set by TME, the possibility that CJD is caused by occasional exposure to scrapie has been intensively studied ever since the transmissibility of CJD was demonstrated in 1968. A large number of investigations have failed to show any epidemiological link between scrapie and CJD. For example, the occurrence of CJD throughout the world is largely independent of the distribution of scrapie and the consumption of sheep products. In addition, several studies have analysed the incidence of CJD in relation to eating habits (e.g. brain), environment (e.g. urban or rural) and various occupations such as those of shepherd, butcher and veterinarian. These studies have also failed to establish a link between scrapie and CJD. It is clear therefore that sheep and goats are not the major reservoir of CJD infection and no other animal reservoir has been identified.

These findings are important in assessing the public health consequences of BSE. Indeed, BSE will be no more of a threat to public health than scrapie unless it is different in the particular ways discussed under The problem (p. 50).

Chapter 1

Geographical distribution

UNITED KINGDOM

BSE was first recognized in the United Kingdom and it is only there that a large-scale epidemic has occurred. By the end of 1990 well over 20 000 cases of BSE had been confirmed in England, Scotland and Wales. The incidence of herds with at least one confirmed case was about 10 percent and the incidence within affected herds was approximately two cases per 100 adults per annum. The overall annual incidence was four cases per 1 000 adults. In Northern Ireland, the total number of BSE cases was around 150. Table 2 gives figures up to the middle of June 1991.

The epidemic started simultaneously in several parts of the country (see Fig. 1) and cases have been distributed over a wide area and in every county ever since (Wilesmith, 1991). The disease occurs predominantly in dairy herds (see The vehicle of infection, p. 20).

TABLE 2

Cumulative total number of histologically confirmed cases of BSE in various countries up to 14 June 1991

United Kingdom	29 907
Northern Ireland	203
Republic of Ireland	39
Switzerland	5
France	4
Oman	2*
Falkland Islands	1*

* All cases in Oman and the Falkland Islands occurred in cattle imported from the United Kingdom.
Source: MAFF, UK.

However, there is marked regional variation in the occurrence of BSE, with a preponderance of cases in the south and east. At the end of 1989 about half of all cases had occurred in just seven counties in the southwest. This

FIGURE 1
Geographical distribution of the first suspected cases of BSE (April 1985 to December 1986)

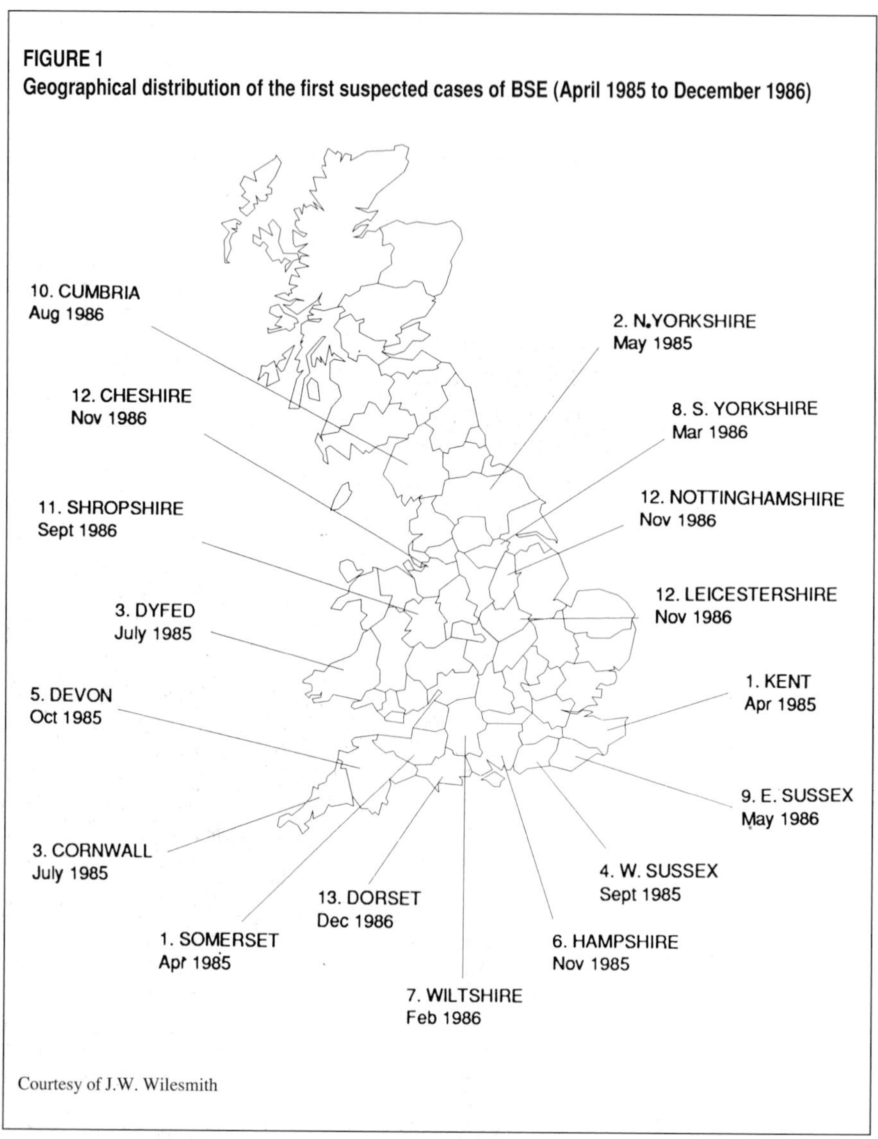

Courtesy of J.W. Wilesmith

pattern is simply a reflection of the number of dairy herds at risk (Matthews, 1990).

The proportion of dairy herds with BSE also shows marked regional variation. In the period from November 1986 (when BSE was first recognized) to July 1989 the percentage of dairy herds with at least one confirmed case

FIGURE 2
Cumulative proportion of dairy herds with BSE in home-bred cattle (November 1986 to August 1990)

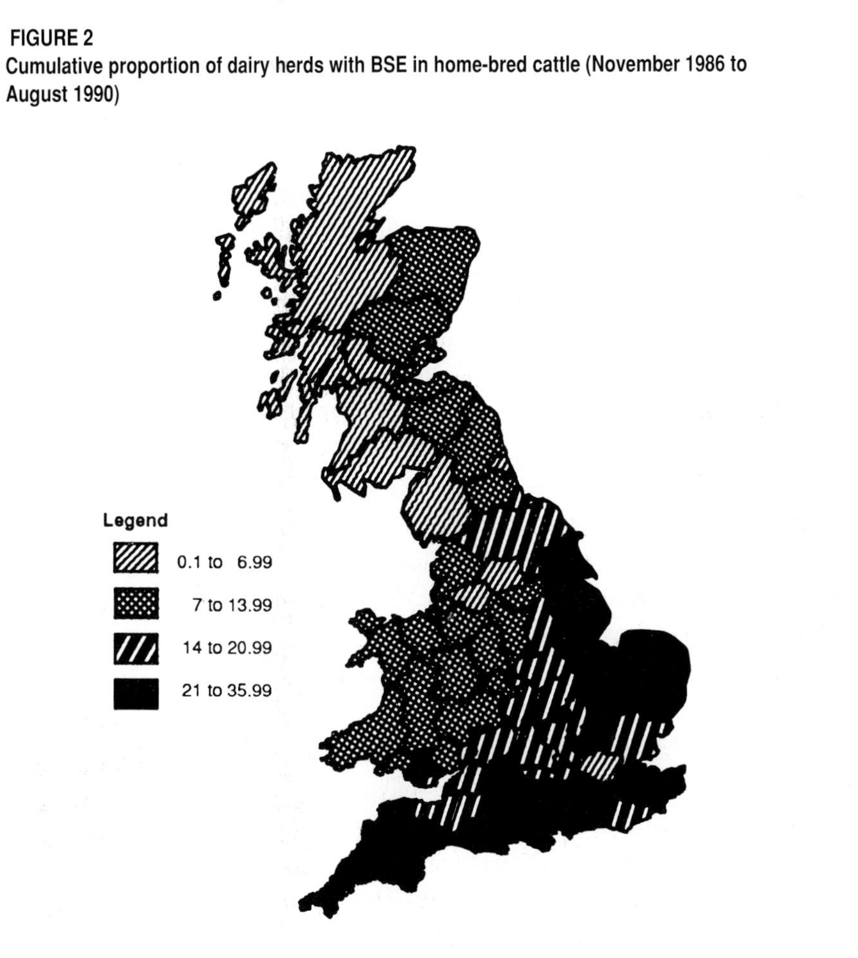

Courtesy of J.W. Wilesmith

of BSE was 12.6 percent in the south, 3.9 percent in the Midlands, 2.8 percent in the north of England and 1.8 percent in Scotland (Wilesmith, Ryan and Atkinson, 1991). Figure 2 gives a more up-to-date pattern which indicates a geographical variation in the exposure of cattle to infection. Epidemiological studies have provided explanations for this variation (see The north-south gradient, p. 24).

OTHER COUNTRIES

Table 2 shows that several cases of BSE have occurred in the Republic of Ireland (Basset and Sheridan, 1989). Some of these were associated with the importation of live animals or meat and bone meal from the United Kingdom. Although scrapie is also present in the Republic, and large amounts of meat and bone meal are produced there, not much is fed to Irish cattle. It is unclear whether any cases of BSE in the country are due to locally produced meat and bone meal.

Two cases of BSE have occurred in Jersey cows in Oman (Carolan, Wells and Wilesmith, 1990). These animals were part of a consignment of 14 pregnant heifers imported from England in 1985. The heifers were born on the same farm in 1983 and investigations into their feeding history suggest exposure to infection during calfhood, before export. The herd of origin has also experienced cases of BSE (Wilesmith, personal communication). Likewise, BSE has occurred in the Falkland Islands in an animal imported from the United Kingdom.

The first case of BSE in continental Europe was reported in November 1990 in a six-year-old Holstein cross that was born and reared in Switzerland (Anon., 1990a). There have subsequently been other Swiss cases (see Table 2). Meat and bone meal had been fed to these animals, but its origin is not known. Switzerland has small populations of sheep and goats. Scrapie has been recorded in a goat but not in sheep.

A case of BSE in Brittany was announced by the French authorities in February 1991 (Anon., 1991a), followed by several other cases (see Table 2). A feed source of infection is suspected. The infection may have been imported or it could have originated in France, a country with a large sheep population and endemic scrapie in several regions.

Chapter 2

Economic implications

The economic consequences of BSE in the United Kingdom have been considerable. To begin with, the only losses due to BSE were those associated with the death or slaughter, on humane grounds, of BSE-affected animals. These losses were borne by individual farmers until August 1988, when a slaughter policy with part compensation was introduced (HMSO, 1988b; 1988c). As the number of BSE cases increased, and more farmers were experiencing a second case, full compensation up to a ceiling was introduced in February 1990 (HMSO, 1990a). In 1989 over 8 000 suspected and confirmed cases of BSE were slaughtered. About 70 percent of the slaughtered animals were disposed of by incineration and the rest by burial at approved sites. The compensation costs for the year were over £2.8 million and the disposal costs amounted to £1.6 million (Matthews, 1990).

Once the epidemiological studies had identified meat and bone meal as the vehicle of infection (see p. 20), the United Kingdom Government banned the feeding of all ruminant-derived protein to ruminants, in July 1988 (HMSO, 1988a). This had an immediate impact on the rendering industry in terms of reduced exports and domestic sales of meat and bone meal. Another effect in the United Kingdom was to increase the costs to abattoirs of animal waste disposal. Subsequently, complex changes in the economics of beef and beef products have been experienced by many sections of the community including producers, retailers and consumers.

The international trade in live cattle was adversely affected when it was realized that some exported animals might have been infected in the United Kingdom before the ruminant protein ban came into effect (July 1988). The following year (July 1989) the Commission of the European Communities (CEC) banned the importation, from the United Kingdom, of all live cattle born before July 1988 (CEC, 1989). A later amendment restricted these exports to calves under six months of age (CEC, 1990a)(see p. 45). Many countries outside the European Economic Community (EEC) have gone further and banned the importation of all live cattle from the United Kingdom. Some have also banned the importation of milk and milk products, despite recommendations to the contrary (OIE, 1990; 1992).

BSE has also had economic consequences in the human and pet food industries. In the winter of 1989/90, the United Kingdom Government banned the use for human food of certain specified bovine offals which potentially contain relatively high titres of BSE infectivity (HMSO, 1989b). This was introduced as a precautionary measure to ensure that the risks to public health from BSE were kept to a minimum regardless of the extent and future course of the epidemic in cattle (see p. 50). The same specified offals were subsequently banned from use in feedstuffs for all mammals and birds, including pets (HMSO, 1990b; see p. 53).

Each of the measures relating to food was tailored to achieve scientifically defined objectives, all of them precautionary in nature. However, they have not prevented several countries from banning imports of a much wider range of human and animal food products containing bovine tissues other than the proscribed offals. This has seriously disrupted the United Kingdom export trade.

Chapter 3
Aetiology

EVIDENCE FOR INFECTION

The aetiology of BSE has never been much in question. BSE is a neurological disease with distinctive microscopic lesions in the central nervous system, exactly like scrapie (see Histopathology, p. 33). Historically, the recognition of the characteristic scrapie-like picture in other diseases led to the studies which demonstrated the experimental transmissibility of TME, kuru, CJD and chronic wasting disease (CWD) (see Table 1). It seemed almost certain that BSE would also be transmissible.

Extracts of BSE-affected brain contain abnormal fibrils very similar to SAF. These fibrils are derived from a normal host-coded protein, PrP, which has undergone an abnormal post-translational modification. The fibrils obtained from BSE-affected brain are made up of the same modified host protein (see Molecular pathology, p. 35). The presence of SAF is another characteristic feature of the transmissible spongiform encephalopathies which indicated an infectious aetiology for BSE.

Because of the long incubation period of these diseases, formal proof of transmissibility came about two years after BSE was first recognized.

The transmissibility of BSE was first demonstrated in mice in which a disease very like murine scrapie developed about 300 days after the combined intracerebral and intraperitoneal injection of affected cattle brain homogenates (Fraser *et al.*, 1988). The same material was injected both intracerebrally and intravenously into cattle and produced cases of BSE after 500 to 650 days (Dawson, Wells and Parker, 1990; Dawson *et al.*, 1991).

Other studies showed that BSE can be transmitted to mice by feeding BSE-affected cattle brain (Barlow and Middleton, 1990a; 1990b), thus reproducing what the epidemiological studies show to be the natural route of transmission in cattle (see The vehicle of infection, p. 20). Studies initiated in 1979, for reasons unconnected with BSE, provide some direct evidence for the transmissibility of scrapie to cattle by the injection of infected brain from cases of experimental scrapie in sheep and goats (Gibbs *et al.*, 1990). There is no doubt that BSE is caused by a scrapie-like infectious agent after long incubation periods.

NATURE OF THE INFECTIOUS AGENT

The physicochemical nature of the scrapie agent is a subject of enduring fascination and considerable controversy. From a practical point of view, knowledge of the chemical structure of the agent would be of enormous importance in providing a diagnostic test of infection. In the absence of sufficient knowledge (and a test), little can be said which is of relevance to the animal health problems posed by BSE. The following is a very brief summary of current information and hypotheses on the nature of the agent which are discussed more fully elsewhere (Kimberlin, 1990a)

Most information has come from studies of the scrapie agent. The agent is small enough to pass through bacteriological filters, thus demonstrating that it is virus-like or subviral in size. But the agent has other properties which are atypical of viruses. The first is that infectivity is highly resistant to many physicochemical treatments, such as heat, and exposure to ionizing or ultra violet radiation. It is no surprise that some infectivity can survive rendering processes (see The vehicle of infection, p. 20, and The start of the BSE epidemic, p. 22). Second, scrapie infection neither induces an immune response nor impairs the immunological responsiveness of the host to other infections. This is in keeping with the non-inflammatory nature of the central nervous system lesions and it is a major reason why there are no laboratory diagnostic tests for the infectious agent. The combination of long incubation period, unusual stability and immunological neutrality explains why the scrapie group of agents have long been known as the "unconventional slow viruses".

There are still major uncertainties about the chemical nature of the scrapie agent. Part of the problem is that studies are critically dependent on bio-assays of infectivity in laboratory animals such as hamsters and mice, with the attendant long incubation periods. But the greatest problem has been the inherent "stickiness" of the scrapie agent which has bedevilled attempts at purification and impeded its chemical characterization.

Ignorance about the structure of the scrapie agent has not prevented other research which has led to a good understanding of the biological properties of the agent, the pathogenesis of the disease and the underlying reasons for its long incubation periods.

Many different strains of scrapie can be identified by their incubation periods, under standard conditions of experimental infection, and by the severity and distribution of histological lesions in the central nervous system. About ten different strains of scrapie are easily recognized by their biological properties in mice and at least three have been identified in hamsters. Mutation of the scrapie agent is well documented in both hamsters and mice and it is clearly not a rare event.

Therefore, scrapie closely resembles other microbial infections in exhibiting strain variation and mutation. This means that the infectious agent has a strain-specific genome. On a priori grounds, the genome is likely to be nucleic acid, even though it has not yet been identified. Some authors maintain that the agent is probably a virus, however unconventional it may be.

The ultraviolet irradiation properties of the scrapie agent indicate that the putative nucleic acid genome is very small. Its estimated target size to ionizing radiation is less than a molecular weight of 100 000. This may be too small for it to code for the protein which, as studies with proteases have shown, is a necessary component of the infectious agent. This has given rise to the "virino" hypothesis which proposes that the protein needed to protect the genome is host-coded. The lack of an immune response to infection could then be explained simply by the absence of foreign antigens. Taxonomically this places virinos between conventional viruses and viroids (a class of plant pathogens which neither need nor code for proteins to be infectious).

The purification of SAF is associated with the partial copurification of infectivity. However, a large amount of modified PrP accumulates in clinically affected brains and it is not easy to prove that the association of infectivity with purified SAF is other than a fortuitous consequence of a very sticky agent. Even if some modified PrP is a component of the infectious agent, there is evidence that much of it is not.

Nevertheless, the association between infectivity and modified PrP has led to further speculation. One possibility is that modified PrP may be the host protein which, according to the virino hypothesis, protects the putative nucleic acid genome. This hypothesis is intellectually attractive because it immediately provides a basis for the interaction between the sip/PrP gene and the infectious agent in natural scrapie.

However, modified PrP is the only molecule to have been identified in preparations containing high infectivity, and another possibility, the "prion" hypothesis, is that modified PrP is itself the infectious agent.

The central issue is the nature of the scrapie genome; on this depends a diagnostic test for infection. Supporters of the virus and virino hypotheses are waiting for a scrapie-specific nucleic acid to be found. Proponents of prions need evidence to explain how scrapie strain variation and mutation can be based on a post-translationally modified, normal protein.

Chapter 4
Epidemiology

BSE was first recognized in November 1986. Retrospective analysis of case histories indicated that a small number of BSE cases had occurred as far back as April 1985. As the result of extensive surveillance, about 130 cases of BSE had been confirmed in the United Kingdom by the end of 1987 (Matthews,1990). Over 2 000 cases were confirmed in 1988, but it should be remembered that BSE became a notifiable disease in June of that year (HMSO, 1988a) and the number of reported cases increased dramatically, from around 60 cases a month to 50 to 60 cases a week, after notification had been introduced. During 1989, the first full year of BSE notification, over 7 000 confirmed cases were recorded. By the end of 1990 the total for the United Kingdom was over 20 000.

EARLY FINDINGS

A major epidemiological study was started in June 1987 (Wilesmith *et al.*, 1988). Although infection was undoubtedly the cause of BSE, it was important to eliminate other possibilities, particularly as the transmissibility of BSE had not yet been demonstrated.

There was no association of the time of onset of BSE with the stage of pregnancy or with calendar month, as might occur following the seasonal use of various pharmaceutical products or agricultural chemicals. Many products were specifically excluded as causes of BSE: for example, vaccines, hormones, organophosphorus fly sprays, synthetic pyrethroid sprays, anthelmintics, herbicides, pesticides, etc. (Wilesmith, 1992).

BSE is clearly not a disease of genetic origin. It has occurred in the majority of United Kingdom dairy breeds and their crosses, in the proportion expected from their representation in the national herd (see Table 3). Analysis of available pedigrees excludes a simple Mendelian pattern of inheritance as the sole cause of the disease.

TABLE 3

Distribution of confirmed cases of BSE in dairy cattle of different breeds and distribution of dairy breeds in the United Kingdom

Breed	Percentage of confirmed BSE cases	Distribution of dairy breeds (%)
Holstein–Friesian	91.5	89.7
Ayrshire	3.9	2.2
Channel Islands	3.7	3.4
Others	0.7	4.7

Source: Wilesmith *et al.*, 1992a.

However, the epidemiological data neither exclude nor support the possibility of bovine genetic factors controlling the susceptibility to an infectious disease, such as occurs with scrapie (Wilesmith *et al.*, 1988; Wijeratne and Curnow, 1990).

But two other pieces of evidence suggest that host genetic variation may not be of great importance in BSE. The first is the remarkably (compared to scrapie) uniform pattern of severity and distribution of vacuolar lesions in BSE (see Histopathology, p. 33). The second is the 100 percent susceptibility and high uniformity of incubation periods seen in a total of 16 Jersey and Holstein-Friesian cattle that had been injected with BSE (Dawson, Wells and Parker, 1990, Dawson *et al.*, 1991). A comparable experiment with scrapie in sheep would have given variability of both incidence and incubation period.

The epidemiological studies further showed that the occurrence of BSE was not associated with the importation of cattle, the use of semen, or the movement of breeding animals between herds. In view of the subsequent evidence that infection with scrapie was the cause of BSE, it was particularly important to find that BSE was not associated with the presence of sheep on the same farms (Wilesmith *et al.*, 1988).

FIGURE 3
Number of cases of BSE by the month and year of onset of clinical signs (April 1985 to April 1991)

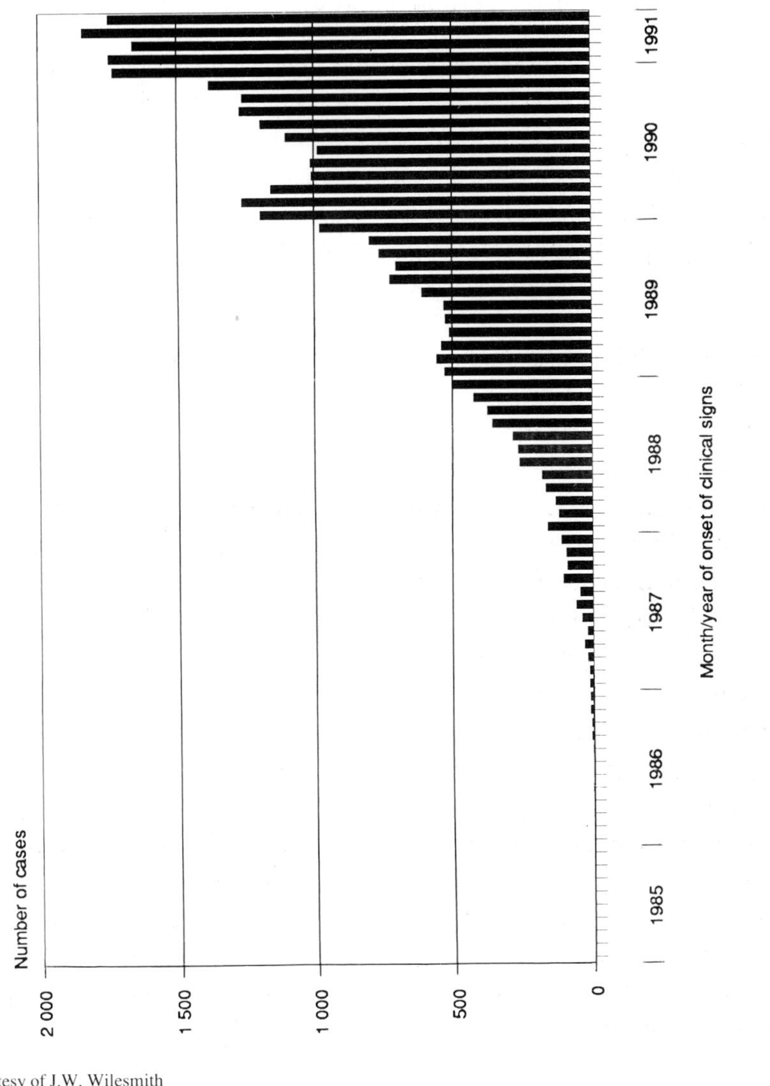

Courtesy of J.W. Wilesmith

THE VEHICLE OF INFECTION

The form of the epidemic curve (showing the occurrence of BSE by month and year of clinical onset) is typical of that of an extended common-source epidemic (see Fig. 3). By a process of elimination, the only common factor to be identified was the feeding of proprietary feedstuffs. Commercial calf pellets, cow cake or protein supplements to home mixed rations have been fed to all cases for which accurate records are available (Wilesmith *et al.*, 1988). This was still true at the end of 1990, when over 20 000 cases of BSE had occurred. Every case is a primary case and there is no evidence of cattle-to-cattle transmission of infection (apart from a report in March 1991 [Anon., 1991b] of a possible instance of maternal transmission to an animal that was born in November 1988, four months after the ruminant protein ban).

Two animal-derived products may be incorporated into proprietary feedstuffs: tallow, and meat and bone meal. The balance of evidence shows meat and bone meal to be the vehicle of infection.

First, the physicochemical properties of the scrapie agent make it more likely to partition with the protein fraction than with the lipids of tallow.

Second, although BSE has shown a wide geographical pattern of occurrence throughout the epidemic, there has always been a striking north-south gradient, with the greater number of cases occurring in the south and east. The basis of this pattern (see The north-south gradient, p.24) is likely to be due to meat and bone meal because both its distribution and incorporation into animal feeds occur within a relatively short distance from its production. Just the opposite is true of tallow (Wilesmith *et al.*, 1988).

The food-borne hypothesis is strongly supported by several other important features of the epidemic (Wilesmith *et al.*, 1988; 1992a; Wilesmith, Ryan and Hueston, 1992c). First, BSE occurs much more often in dairy herds than in beef suckler herds. The difference is not related to any variation in breed susceptibility but to different feeding practices. In dairy herds, it is common to feed concentrates containing meat and bone meal during the first six months of life. Such feeds are rarely used for beef suckler calves, whose food consists of milk from the dam, mostly supplemented by conserved forage and cereals. About 85 percent of all BSE cases in beef suckler herds

TABLE 4

Cumulative proportion of herds with BSE in home-bred cattle according to type and size of herd

Herd type	Herd size				Total
	< 50	50-99	100-199	>199	
Dairy and mixed					
No. of BSE herds	779	2 384	2 615	424	6 263
No. of herds at risk	21 072	15 728	6 935	1 032	44 767
Percentage affected	3.70	15.16	37.71	41.09	13.99
Beef suckler					
No. of BSE herds	77	40	20	4	142
No. of herds at risk	48 182	4 454	1 347	183	54 166
Percentage affected	0.16	0.90	1.48	2.19	0.26

Note: Total includes 61 dairy herds and one beef herd of unknown size.
Source: Wilesmith *et al.*, 1992a.

occur in purchased animals and a high proportion of these are cross-bred animals that were born in dairy herds and probably infected there before being sold. A comparison of BSE incidence in herds with only home-bred cases shows that the proportion of dairy herds affected is about 50 times greater than the proportion of beef suckler herds affected (see Table 4).

Second, the incidence of BSE-affected herds of either type increases progressively with herd size; the bigger the herd, the more feed is required and the greater the chances of buying an infected batch (see Table 4). Third, over 50 percent of all affected herds have had only one case and another 20 percent have had only two. Both observations strongly indicate a low average exposure to a source of infection outside the cattle population.

Finally, a case-control study shows that the inclusion of meat and bone meal in proprietary calf feeds is a statistically significant risk factor for the occurrence of BSE (Wilesmith, Ryan and Hueston, 1992c). A computer-based simulation model has been constructed to analyse some of the time scales of the epidemic (Wilesmith *et al.*, 1988). The model shows that the exposure of the cattle population must have started abruptly, around the winter of 1981/82. Both adults and calves have been exposed but the majority of affected animals were exposed as calves. This means that the age-specific incidences will reflect incubation period.

Since the incubation period was originally estimated to range from 2.5 to at least eight years, the model predicts that, during the earlier years of the epidemic, more and more cases will occur in older animals as the full effect of the incubation period distribution becomes manifest. This prediction is confirmed by the observation of a higher incidence of BSE in animals aged five years and above in 1988 than in 1987 (Wilesmith, Ryan and Atkinson, 1991; Wilesmith *et al*., 1992a).

As of July 1991, the incidence of BSE was highest in four- and five-year-olds. The oldest recorded case was 15 years and the youngest was 22 months (but born before the ruminant protein ban was introduced).

THE START OF THE BSE EPIDEMIC

A key epidemiological finding is that exposure to a scrapie-like agent, sufficient to cause clinical disease, started in the winter of 1981/82.

It seems likely that the epidemic began by the infection of cattle with scrapie agent from sheep. However, the present epidemiological evidence does not distinguish between this and an alternative possibility, namely that an endemic infection of cattle existed long before the current epidemic started, but was undetected because the incidence of clinical disease was so low. To be realistic, the incidence would have had to be less than one case per 100 000 adult cattle per annum, which was the incidence at the very start of the epidemic (Wilesmith *et al*., 1988). Such a possibility has been suggested as the cause of an outbreak of TME on a ranch in the United States where mink were regularly fed dead cattle (Marsh *et al*., 1991). Undetected BSE could exist in other countries but, until there is direct evidence for such a possibility, it must be assumed that scrapie was the original cause of BSE.

It is well established that scrapie can be experimentally transmitted, both within and between species, by the feeding or intragastric administration of infected material (Kimberlin, 1990a). Scrapie has been endemic in the United Kingdom for nearly three centuries, and the country also has a very large sheep population. In terms of animal waste, about 15 percent of all rendered material is ovine compared with about 45 percent of bovine origin (HMSO, 1985). But if a large sheep population (relative to cattle) with endemic scrapie, and the use of meat and bone meal as a feed supplement, are necessary preconditions for BSE, why did the disease not occur before the 1980s?

During the production of meat and bone meal, the temperatures achieved by most rendering processes operating at normal atmospheric pressure would not be high enough to guarantee the total elimination of large amounts of scrapie infectivity (Taylor, 1989a). Yet they may have been adequate to disinfect lower levels of contamination, until recent changes in rendering processes allowed sufficient infection to survive in meat and bone meal (Wilesmith, Ryan and Atkinson, 1991).

A detailed investigation has been carried out on the 46 rendering plants in operation in the United Kingdom in 1988 (Wilesmith, Ryan and Atkinson, 1991).

During the period from 1972 to 1988, the proportion of meat and bone meal produced by continuous processes, as opposed to batch processes, increased from 0 percent to about 75 percent. However, this is unlikely to have been a major factor in causing BSE, for two reasons. First, the change was too gradual to account for the sudden onset of exposure of cattle in 1981/82. Second, the survey did not reveal a difference in the mean maximum temperatures between continuous and batch processes. In addition, the particle size of the raw material is smaller in the continuous processes: this would favour a more, not less, efficient inactivation of scrapie.

The same period (1972-1988) also witnessed a decline in the use of solvent extraction, which was employed to increase the yield of tallow. But this change was quite abrupt. The proportion of meat and bone meal produced by the use of solvents decreased by nearly 50 percent between 1980 and 1983. Not only does this fit the predicted onset of exposure but the move away from solvent extraction would have meant the loss of two partial scrapie-inactivation steps.

It is likely that the usual conditions of solvent extraction, for about eight hours at 70° C, would have reduced infectivity and/or made the residual infectivity more heat sensitive. The second step was the direct application of superheated steam to meat and bone meal for 15 to 30 minutes to remove the last traces of solvent. Wet heating is much more effective against scrapie than dry heating (Wilesmith, Ryan and Atkinson, 1991). It can be concluded that the cessation of solvent extraction was a major factor causing BSE.

THE NORTH-SOUTH GRADIENT

Only two rendering plants in the United Kingdom still use solvent extraction, and both are in Scotland. This helps to explain the much lower incidence of BSE in Scotland (see Fig. 2).

In addition, half of the remaining plants produce greaves as an intermediate product which is then sold to other plants for further processing to produce meat and bone meal. Some of the greaves is mixed with raw material and subjected to a complete processing cycle. About 15 percent of all meat and bone meal receives this second heat treatment.

However, there are major regional differences in the amount of reprocessing of greaves. Very little meat and bone meal is produced in this way in the south of England, but increasing proportions are produced in the Midlands, the north of England and Scotland. This variation would contribute to the north-south gradient in the incidence of BSE (Wilesmith, Ryan and Atkinson, 1991).

Other factors could also be involved. Although both sheep and scrapie are widely distributed in the United Kingdom, some regional variation would be expected in the amount of infected sheep material entering different rendering plants. There would also be variation in the use of meat and bone meal by different commercial compounders of cattle feedstuffs, as well as differences in their geographical market share of sales.

Present epidemiological studies seek to evaluate these factors. However, the situation in much of the country is complex (Wilesmith *et al.*, 1992a) and a more fruitful approach has been to focus on BSE in Northern Ireland (Denny *et al.*, 1991) and the Channel Islands. It is interesting that the dramatically different occurrences of BSE in Guernsey and Jersey can be associated with differences in the manufacturers supplying feedstuffs from the mainland (Wilesmith, 1992).

THE RECYCLING OF INFECTION IN CATTLE

There is now sufficient information to reconstruct the salient events in the BSE epidemic in the United Kingdom.

As explained above, it is now assumed that scrapie was the original cause of the BSE epidemic. It is theoretically possible that BSE originated with a mutant scrapie strain that arose spontaneously in sheep and simply happened to be more pathogenic for cattle than other scrapie strains. This possibility is discounted by the form of the epidemic, which would require the simultaneous emergence of this mutant strain in many flocks throughout the country (see Fig. 1). This is improbable (Wilesmith *et al.*, 1988). It is far more likely that the epidemic was started by one scrapie strain that is common in different breeds of sheep, or possibly, a few strains that behaved in a similar manner when crossing the sheep-to-cattle species barrier.

However, the continued exposure of cattle to sheep scrapie was not the ultimate driving force of the epidemic. On the contrary, the epidemic would inevitably have been amplified by the subsequent recycling, via meat and bone meal, of infected cattle material within the cattle population. Recycling would have produced the equivalent of a serial passage of the infection, as happened with kuru. Because of the length of BSE incubation periods, recycling would have established the pattern of the epidemic long before BSE was even recognized (see The development of the epidemic, p. 26).

One consequence of recycling is that it would favour the selection of cattle-adapted strains of agent, and these strains could differ from those in the sheep population. Present evidence suggests little or no allelic variation in any cattle genes that might affect the incubation period. This means that all cattle would tend to exert a similar selective pressure, favouring strains with the shortest incubation period. Since some scrapie strains are known to be more heat stable than others, the rendering process itself could also have exerted a uniform selective pressure favouring heat-resistant strains.

Several isolates of the BSE agent are being studied by experimental passage in mice (Fraser *et al.*, 1988; Fraser, Bruce and McConnell, 1991). Preliminary evidence shows that BSE isolates from geographically separate sources have strikingly similar incubation periods and other properties. This suggests that BSE was caused by a single common scrapie strain in sheep.

This strain could have been selected and passaged unchanged in cattle (through recycling). Alternatively, it could have given rise to a mutant strain in cattle that was subsequently selected because it had a shorter incubation period in cattle than the parental strain.

The latter possibility is somewhat favoured by the evidence that isolates of BSE, while strikingly similar to one another, are different from past isolates of sheep scrapie in mice and also from one recent scrapie isolate (Fraser, Bruce and McConnell, 1991). Unfortunately, natural scrapie isolates that were contemporary with the start of the exposure of cattle are not available to make the most appropriate comparison.

THE DEVELOPMENT OF THE EPIDEMIC

With experimental scrapie, serial passage in a new species usually involves a reduction of incubation period, even when there is no selection of strains. In addition, strain selection always favours the strain with the shortest incubation period (Kimberlin, Cole and Walker, 1987; Kimberlin, Walker and Fraser, 1989). Therefore, a likely consequence of the recycling of BSE in cattle is a reduction in incubation period (and this would be independent of any reduction resulting from an increase in infectivity, as discussed below). Evidence of a reduced incubation period is being sought by analysing the age at onset of disease, which reflects incubation period, as a function of year of birth, which is when a majority of cases would have been exposed (Wilesmith and Ryan, personal communication).

The second consequence of recycling is the multiplication of infectivity during each passage. This would increase the total amount of infectivity circulating in the cattle population. The third consequence is that there is no longer a species barrier. In terms of effective dose, this could be the most important consequence because the species barrier is usually the limiting factor in the interspecies transmission of scrapie-like agents. The epidemic would inevitably be driven by cattle BSE, which would then have a selective advantage over sheep scrapie.

A change in effective dose is reflected in the stepwise increase in the incidence of BSE, starting in mid-1989 (see Fig. 3). This change is unlikely to be due to an increased ascertainment of cases, which would have reached a consistent high level by this stage of the epidemic. Moreover, the same change was observed in the Channel Islands, where the reporting of cases has always been close to 100 percent (Wilesmith *et al.*, 1992a). Therefore, the increase of BSE in mid-1989 suggests a substantial degree of recycling of infected cattle material around 1984/85 (Wilesmith and Wells, 1991).

The way in which the incidence of BSE increased is particularly interesting. One would expect a higher effective dose to increase both the number of affected herds and the incidence within affected herds. In practice, the latter has changed little, but there has been a large increase in the number of herds with BSE. This means that the average dose of infectivity was extremely low and the main effect of recycling was to increase the *number* of batches of meat and bone meal with the minimum "threshold" amount of infectivity necessary to infect cattle, rather than the *concentration* of infectivity within batches. Later on, one might expect the average concentration to have risen sufficiently to cause a more obvious increase in the incidence of BSE within affected herds (Wilesmith, personal communication).

Up to July 1991 about 70 percent of all affected herds had only had one or two cases. This is in marked contrast to some outbreaks of TME in which morbidity approached 100 percent. The tragedy of BSE is that, despite the low exposure, a substantial proportion of a large cattle population (about four million adults) was exposed from 1981/82 until the summer of 1988 when the ruminant protein ban came into effect. This explains why the total number of BSE cases in the United Kingdom is so high.

It is difficult to estimate the attack rate for BSE because the distribution of infectious agent in meat and bone meal would not have been homogeneous and feeding regimes would have varied from herd to herd and from year to year.

However, the theoretical approach discussed by Wilesmith (1991) gives some idea of the attack rate. If the average dairy herd has 70 adult cows and the annual replacement rate is 20 percent, then each new birth cohort joining the adult herd would comprise 14 heifers. A single case in the cohort thus represents an attack rate of 7 percent (Wilesmith, 1991).

The most important remaining question is the future course of the epidemic. This is discussed in Chapter 9.

SPONGIFORM ENCEPHALOPATHY IN OTHER ANIMAL SPECIES

The epidemiology of BSE shows how animals can be exposed to scrapie infection via processed feedstuffs, not just by the feeding of untreated sheep carcasses or offal as was indicated by studies of TME.

Prior to BSE, a transmissible spongiform encephalopathy known as chronic wasting disease (CWD) (see Table 1) was described in captive mule deer *(Odocoileus hemionus hemionus)* and Rocky Mountain elk *(Cervus elaphus nelsoni)* held in wildlife facilities in Colorado and Wyoming (Kimberlin, 1990a). About 100 cases have been diagnosed since 1967 (Williams *et al.*, 1990). The majority of affected animals were born in the wild and found as orphans. A source of infection in captivity has not been identified. Scrapie occurs in the United States and an exogenous feed source of infection is a possibility. However, cases of disease have been diagnosed in free-ranging deer and elk (Williams *et al.*, 1990).

Concurrently with the BSE epidemic in the United Kingdom, cases of spongiform encephalopathy have occurred in five exotic species of ruminants kept in wildlife parks and zoos in England. The species are:

- nyala *(Tragelaphus angasi)* in 1986 (Jeffrey and Wells, 1988);
- gemsbok *(Oryx gazella)* in 1987 (Jeffrey and Wells, 1988; Wilesmith *et al.*, 1988);
- Arabian oryx *(Oryx leucoryx)* in 1989 (Kirkwood *et al.*,1990);
- greater kudu *(Tragelaphus strepsiceros)* in 1989 (Kirkwood *et al.*; 1990).
- eland *(Taurotragus oryx)* in 1989 (Fleetwood and Furley, 1990).

The pathology of these diseases leaves no doubt about their nature and likely aetiology. Most, if not all, of the animals involved were fed diets containing meat and bone meal before the ruminant protein ban was instituted. Brain material from clinical cases in a nyala and a greater kudu has produced spongiform encephalopathy after injection into mice.

The diseases in zoo animals differ from BSE in three respects. First, the clinical duration was considerably shorter than in BSE, sometimes just a few days. Second, the incidence of disease in the zoo animals was disproportionately high in relation to the size of the population exposed. Third, the age of onset of clinical disease was much younger (30 to 38 months) in the zoo animals than in cattle. The youngest case of BSE so far recorded is at 22 months, but the onset of clinical signs is typically at four to five years.

These findings suggest a higher effective exposure of the zoo animals than cattle. But the route of exposure and the inclusion rate of meat and bone meal would have been similar. It seems, therefore, that the species barrier was lower for the exotic ungulates, resulting in an increased susceptibility to infection.

A second case in a greater kudu was reported at the end of 1990 (Anon., 1990b). The animal was born in April 1989 and was never fed ruminant protein. Disease developed 19 months later and the clinical duration was only a few days. The calf was born to the first case of spongiform encephalopathy in a greater kudu and the simplest explanation is that it became infected from its mother (Kirkwood *et al.*, 1992). Maternal transmission of infection is well established in sheep scrapie and the possibility of it occurring in cattle should now be considered more likely (see The possibility of endemic infection, p. 55).

Since January 1990 cases of a new spongiform encephalopathy have occurred in several adult domestic cats in various parts of the United Kingdom (Wyatt *et al.*, 1990; 1991; Leggett, Dukes and Pirie, 1990). Feline spongiform encephalopathy (FSE) is experimentally transmissible to mice by the injection of affected brain. As with the zoo animals, it seems likely that FSE was also the result of food-borne infection, but the fact that it was only recognized in early 1990 suggests that the infection may have been BSE rather than scrapie.

Cats are fed a wide variety of different foods, including offals and prepared pet foods containing meat and bone meal. There have been insufficient cases of FSE to identify the source of infection. The total number of cases in 1990 was 12, and only six had occurred in the United Kingdom by the end of July 1991. Because there would be no recycling of infection from cat to cat via feed, a large-scale epidemic like BSE seems unlikely.

Before the first case of FSE had been recognized, the United Kingdom pet food industry had already instituted a voluntary "specified offals ban" in

1989, as a precautionary measure against the infection of cats and other domestic species. This measure became mandatory in 1990 (HMSO, 1990b) (see Minimizing the exposure of other species, p. 53).

Chapter 5

Clinical signs

The original clinical description of BSE was based on the first six cases to be recorded (Wells *et al.*, 1987). Subsequent accounts show that the frequency of different clinical signs has remained constant during the course of the epidemic (Cranwell *et al.*, 1988; Gilmour *et al.*, 1988; Wilesmith *et al.*, 1988; 1992b; Scott *et al.*, 1988; 1989; Winter *et al.*, 1989; Wilesmith and Wells, 1991). The following account is based on the signs recorded in a comprehensive study of nearly 200 cases of BSE (Wilesmith *et al.*, 1988). Supplementary clinical data have now been obtained from the reports of over 17 000 confirmed cases (Wilesmith *et al.*, 1992b).

Cases of BSE show a combination of neurological and general signs of disease. The neurological signs fall into three categories:

- Changes in mental state were observed, most commonly seen as apprehension, frenzy and nervousness when confronted by doorways and other entrances. About 98 percent of all cases showed altered behaviour in this category.
- Abnormalities of posture and movement occurred in 93 percent of cases. The most common manifestations were hind-limb ataxia, tremors and falling.
- Changes in sensation were a feature of about 95 percent of all cases. This was exhibited in many different ways, but the most striking was hyperaesthesia, to both touch and sound.

A large majority of cases (87 percent) exhibited signs that fell into all three neurological categories. This is consistent with a diffuse central nervous system disorder. There are many points of similarity in the clinical signs of scrapie and BSE. The most obvious difference is that pruritus was only seen occasionally in BSE.

In addition, there were some general clinical signs associated with BSE of which the most frequent were loss of body condition (78 percent), live weight loss (73 percent) and reduced milk yield (70 percent). A good appetite was maintained in the great majority of cases. At some stage in the clinical course, about 79 percent of all cases showed one of the above general signs along with signs in each of the three neurological categories. No pathologically confirmed cases of BSE exhibited only general signs.

There is considerable day-to-day variation in the presence and severity of individual signs. Keeping animals in a quiet and familiar environment reduces the severity of some signs, particularly hyperaesthesia. But over a period of weeks, the clinical signs are progressive, leading to recumbency and death. However, the slaughter of the great majority of affected animals becomes necessary at an earlier stage because of unmanageable behaviour and injury from repeated falling.

The duration of the clinical disease, from the earliest signs to death or slaughter, can range from under two weeks to as long as a year. The average period is about one to two months.

Chapter 6
Pathology

BSE resembles other members of the scrapie family in not having any gross pathological lesions consistently associated with disease, nor any biochemical or haematological abnormalities (Aldridge *et al.*, 1988; Johnson and Whitaker,1988; Scott *et al.*, 1988; 1990a). Characteristic histopathological and molecular changes are found in the central nervous system.

HISTOPATHOLOGY

In common with the other diseases in the scrapie family, BSE has a distinctive non-inflammatory pathology with three main features (Wells, Wilesmith and McGill, 1991):

- The most important diagnostic lesion is the presence of bilaterally symmetrical neuronal vacuolation, in processes and in soma. The former consists of a microcystic vacuolation (spongiform change) of the grey matter neuropil (Fig. 4a). This is the major vacuolar lesion of BSE. The other type of vacuolation consists of large, empty spaces distending neuronal perikarya (Fig. 4b). This type of vacuolation is a conspicuous feature of natural scrapie but it is less prominent in BSE. Neurons with somal vacuolation frequently have an otherwise normal appearance. However, scattered necrotic soma are seen and, as with natural scrapie, neuronal loss is an occasional but rarely conspicuous feature.
- Hypertrophy of astrocytes often accompanies vacuolation. This has been demonstrated in routinely stained sections and also in sections immunostained for glial fibrillary acidic protein (Fig. 4c).
- Cerebral amyloidosis is an inconstant histological feature of the scrapie family of diseases. It is present in BSE but mostly as sparse, focal deposits in a small proportion of cases. Congophilic plaques showing characteristic dichroism in polarized light were found in the thalamus of

one out of 20 cases examined systematically for amyloid. The plaques immunostained for PrP (see Molecular pathology).

A number of studies have examined the quantitative distribution of the vacuolar changes in BSE. A study of 22 clinically affected brains (Scott *et al*., 1990b) showed that the mean vacuolar densities were greatest in: the medulla oblongata (in the solitary tract nucleus, the spinal tract nucleus of the trigeminal nerve, vestibular nuclei and the reticular formation); the central grey matter in the midbrain; and the paraventricular area in the hypothalamus, thalamus and the septal area. In contrast, the vacuolar change was often minimal in the cerebellum, hippocampus, cerebral cortex and basal nuclei.

Another quantitative study examined a series of 100 cases, sampled before July 1989 (Wells, Wilesmith and McGill, 1991). The vacuolar patterns in the brain were remarkably uniform in contrast to the variability described in sheep scrapie.

These findings indicate a uniformity in the pathogenesis of BSE in terms

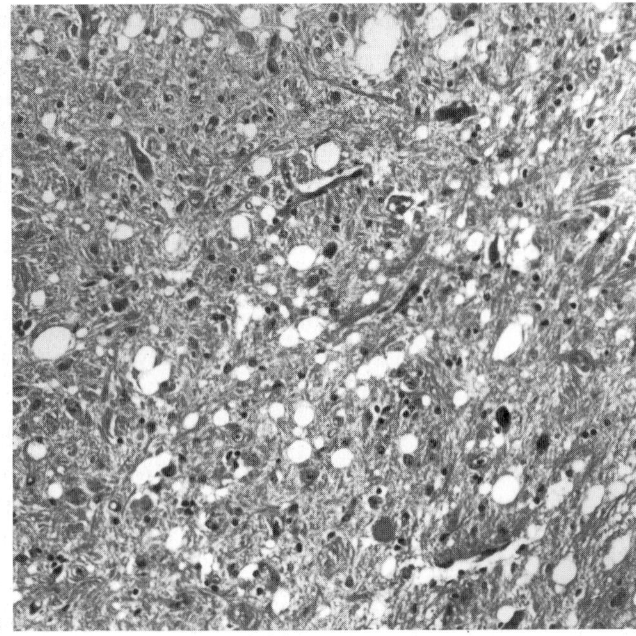

FIGURE 4a
Lesions of BSE: spongiform change in the solitary tract nucleus of the medulla oblongata. Haematoxylin and eosin; X 160

Courtesy of G.A.H. Wells

of the route of infection (through the alimentary tract) and the major strain(s) of the infectious agent in cattle.

Electron microscope (EM) observations on thin sections of BSE-affected brain revealed the expected findings of a scrapie-like disease (Liberski, 1990). These included numerous membrane-bound intracellular vacuoles, predominantly in dendrites. Many dendrites and axons contained accumulations of neurofilaments, mitochondria and electron-dense bodies. In addition, tubulovesicular structures were seen. These are similar to the structures found in scrapie except that those seen in BSE-affected brains were membrane-bound. This might be a distinctive lesion of BSE but it requires further investigation.

MOLECULAR PATHOLOGY

In addition to the histological lesions that characterize the scrapie family of diseases, extracts of clinically affected brains contain an abundance of characteristic abnormal fibrils (SAF) which are readily identified by

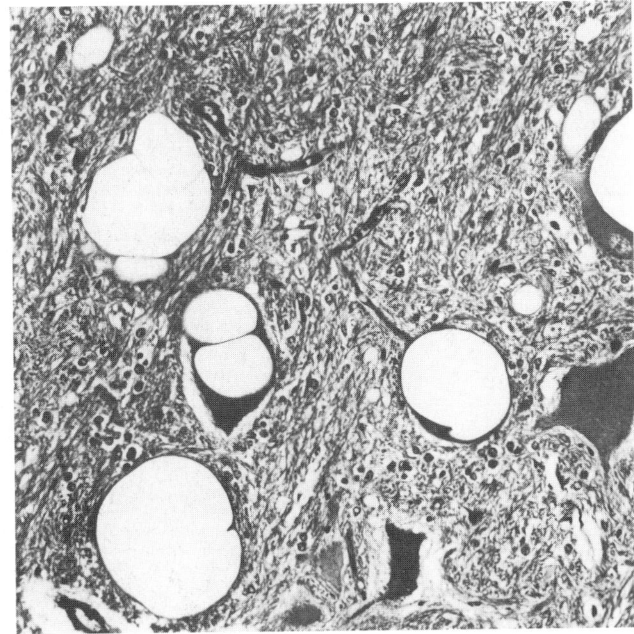

FIGURE 4b
Lesions of BSE: large vacuoles in neuronal perikarya of the vestibular nucleus complex of the medulla oblongata. Haematoxylin and eosin; X 175

Courtesy of G.A.H. Wells

negative stain EM. Their presence in extracts of BSE-affected brain was important in confirming the histological observations that BSE is a scrapie-like disease of cattle (Wells *et al.*, 1987).

SAF are easily purified and much is known about them (Hope *et al.*, 1988). They are derived from a normal (i.e. host-coded) membrane glycoprotein, known as PrP, which is present in many tissues, particularly the brain. In the course of scrapie infection, this normal protein undergoes an abnormal post-translational modification (in ways that are not yet understood) and acquires the ability to form fibrils. The modified protein is partially resistant to proteolytic enzymes so that it accumulates in brain, often to about ten times the concentration of the normal protein.

The fibrils from BSE-affected brain have been purified and studied in terms of size, protease resistance, immunoreactivity (with antibodies prepared against SAF), lectin binding and partial N-terminal amino acid sequence. The results show conclusively that the fibrils from BSE-affected brain are made from bovine PrP (Hope *et al.*, 1988).

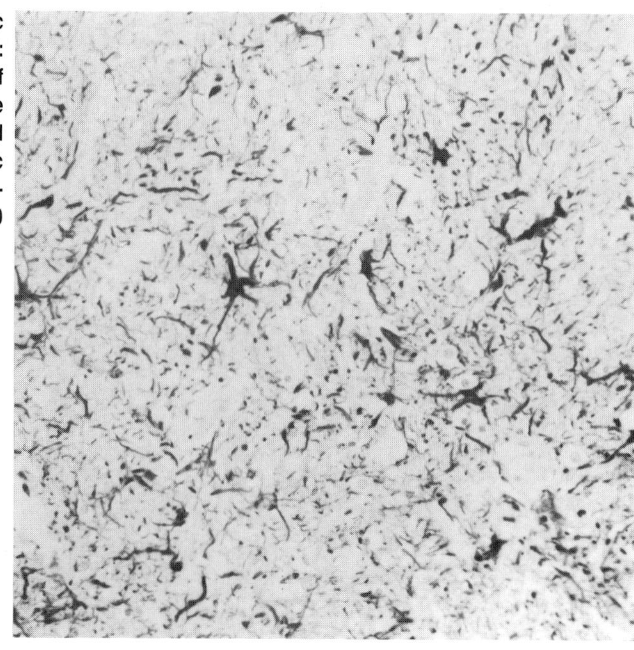

FIGURE 4c
Lesions of BSE: hypertrophy of astrocytes in the gracile nucleus immunostained for glial fibrillary acidic protein, an astrocyte-specific marker; X 250

Courtesy of G.A.H. Wells

There are three ways in which the fibril form of PrP can be detected:

- SAF can be identified by their characteristic morphology when examined by EM (Wells *et al.*, 1987; Hope *et al.*, 1988; Scott *et al.*, 1990b).
- Purified or even crude preparations of SAF can be analysed by western blotting after polyacrylamide gel electrophoresis. This method does not detect SAF (which are dissolved prior to electrophoresis), but the constituent protein, modified PrP. The protease resistance of modified PrP allows it to be distinguished from normal PrP, which is much more sensitive to digestion with proteases (Hope *et al.*, 1988; Scott *et al.*, 1990b).
- The modified form of PrP can be detected in sections of BSE-affected brain by immunocytochemical staining with antibodies to SAF. The primary amino acid sequence of normal PrP is highly conserved in different species so the antibodies do not necessarily have to be raised against SAF purified from affected cattle. Since anti-SAF antibodies recognize normal PrP, this has to be removed by treatment with proteases. Little work of this kind has been published on BSE but it has been shown that the amyloid plaques occasionally seen in brain are immunocytochemically positive for PrP (Wells, Wilesmith and McGill, 1991).

Chapter 7
Diagnosis

There are no routine laboratory diagnostic tests to identify infected cattle before the onset of clinical disease. The diagnosis of BSE therefore depends on the recognition of clinical signs and confirmation by histological examination of the central nervous system. A clinical diagnosis can also be confirmed by EM, biochemical or immunocytochemical detection of SAF or the constituent protein, modified PrP.

CLINICAL SIGNS

The most common presenting sign is nervous behaviour (Fig. 5). This can be seen as a separation from the rest of the herd at pasture, a reluctance to enter the milking parlour and vigorous kicking in response to being milked. The earliest locomotor signs are subtle changes in the hind-limb gait and difficulty in rising from a normal recumbent position.

The early changes in behaviour can be confused with hypomagnesaemia and nervous ketosis. Unresponsiveness to treatment is one way to distinguish these two conditions from BSE. Another is the more insidious onset of the signs of BSE, together with their chronic progression over a period of weeks. The locomotor changes, in particular, progress to an obvious swaying gait, shortened stride and awkwardness in turning.

As mentioned previously, the predominant neurological signs of BSE are apprehension, hyperaesthesia and ataxia (see Fig. 6). Animals exhibiting a combination of these three signs for more than one month should be regarded as likely cases of BSE (Wilesmith *et al.*, 1992b).

With the kind of experience gained by many observers in the United Kingdom, BSE can be diagnosed with a high degree of accuracy. Even so, all suspect cases of BSE in the country are examined by routine histopathology. Histological confirmation is essential whenever the BSE status of an individual animal needs to be established with certainty.

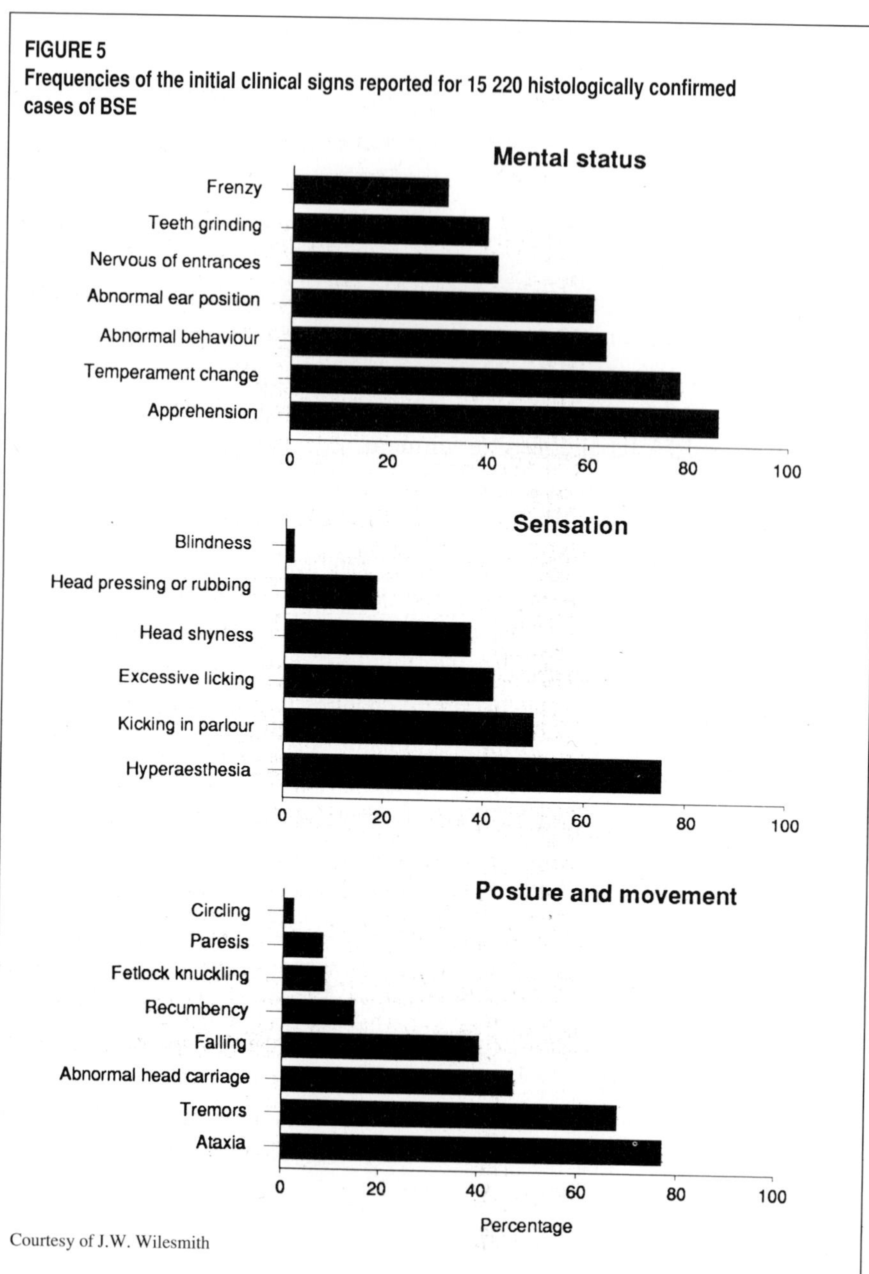

FIGURE 5

Frequencies of the initial clinical signs reported for 15 220 histologically confirmed cases of BSE

Courtesy of J.W. Wilesmith

FIGURE 6
Frequencies of the neurological signs in 17 154 histologically confirmed cases of BSE

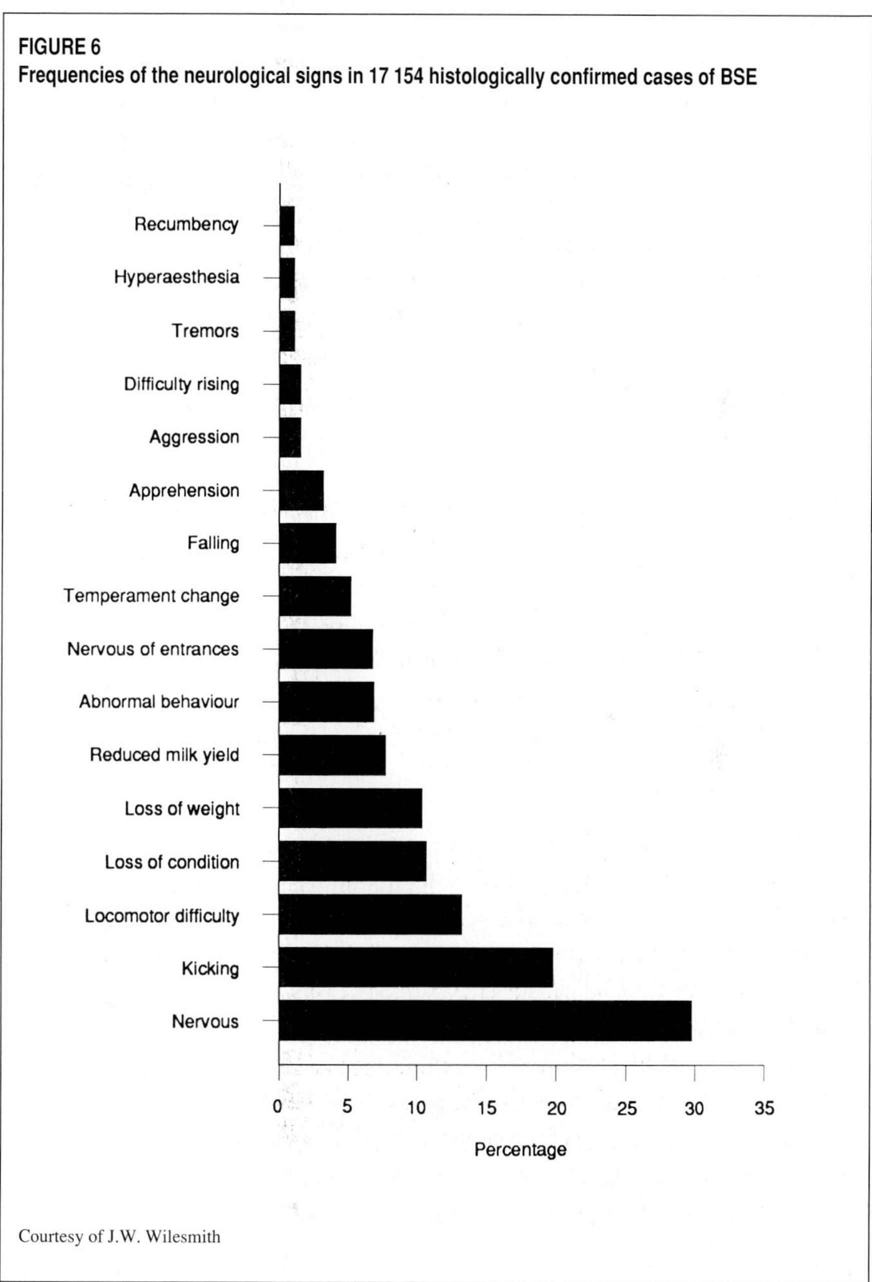

Courtesy of J.W. Wilesmith

HISTOPATHOLOGY

The histopathological diagnosis of BSE can be made on the basis of neuroparenchymal vacuolation in the brains of suspected cases. It should be noted that vacuolation in neuronal perikarya is occasionally seen as an incidental feature in cattle (Wells *et al.*, 1987). The frequency of such "normal" vacuolation is usually very low relative to that associated with clinical disease, and it is largely confined to the red nucleus (see Fig. 7). Artefactual vacuolation can also be produced under certain conditions of histological processing, but this principally affects white matter (Wells and Wells, 1989).

The recognition of BSE as a new disease of cattle was based on the routine examination of coronal sections representing the major brain regions (Wells *et al.*, 1987). This would obviously be the required procedure when presented with a possible case of BSE for the first time.

Later in the epidemic, the consistent presence of pathognomonic lesions in the brain stem justified a simplified examination of just four coronal sections which include parts of the medulla oblongata, pons and mesencephalon. Subsequently, the increasing scale of the epidemic and the requirement for histological examination of all suspected cases created the need (and also provided the material) to develop an even simpler procedure.

A study of 684 bovine brains, including 563 confirmed cases, evaluated the histological diagnosis of BSE by examination of a single section of medulla, routinely taken at the obex (Wells *et al.*, 1989). The high frequency of vacuolar changes in two nuclei in the medulla (the solitary tract nucleus and the spinal tract nucleus of the trigeminal nerve) made it possible to identify 99.6 percent of BSE cases that had been confirmed by the more extensive sampling of the brain. This means that other areas of the brain need only be examined when lesions in the medulla are minimal or absent.

DETECTION OF THE FIBRILLAR FORM OF PrP

The convenience and reliability of brain histology obviates the need to base routine diagnoses of BSE on the detection of modified PrP. However, there are situations when it would be useful. The most obvious is when a suspect case of BSE has arisen unexpectedly and it is imperative to be sure of the diagnosis. In these circumstances, the detection of SAF or modified PrP is a useful adjunct to histopathological diagnosis. It would be indispensable if the brain was unsuitable for histology: for example, if removal or fixation was excessively delayed. The protease resistance of SAF makes it possible to isolate them from brain that has undergone significant autolysis. However, SAF can only be purified satisfactorily from fresh or frozen brain, not fixed brain.

Two systematic studies have evaluated the detection of SAF in the routine diagnosis of BSE (Scott *et al.*, 1990b). In the first, 144 histologically positive BSE brains and 23 negative brains were examined by purification of SAF and detection by EM. There were no false positives (out of 23 brains) but a large proportion of false negatives was observed (53 percent of 144 brains). The reason for the false negatives was that the brain areas selected for assay were suboptimal; they had been chosen after the priority areas for histopathology had been allocated.

A second study, of 22 brains, showed that the number of SAF approxi-

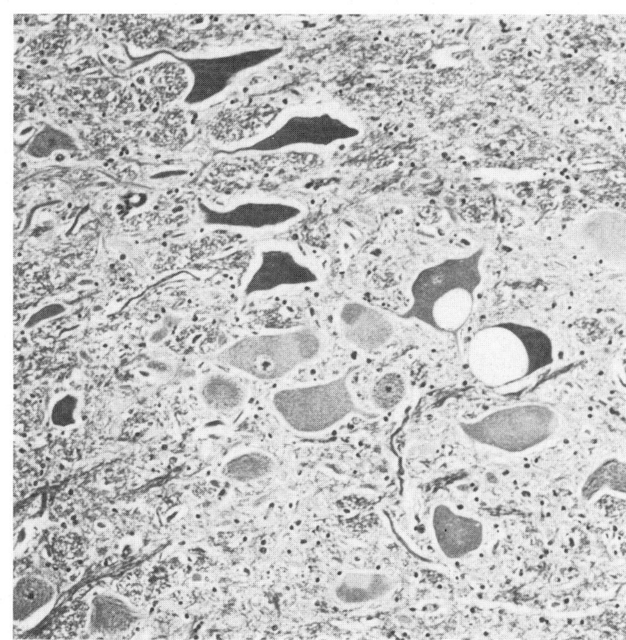

FIGURE 7
Mild vacuolation of neuronal perikarya, in the absence of other neuropathology, in the red nucleus of a clinically normal cow. Haematoxylin andeosin; X 120

Courtesy of G.A.H. Wells

mated the severity of the vacuolar changes. For this second series, fibrils were detected in samples of all 22 BSE cases when brain stem areas were examined. This study also demonstrated the sensitivity of fibril detection by western blotting (Scott *et al.*, 1990b).

Chapter 8
Prevention

It scarcely needs stating that, at present, vaccination is not an appropriate way of preventing any of the diseases in the scrapie family; there is no known protective immune response to infection for a vaccine to enhance. However, BSE is obviously not a highly contagious disease and it can be prevented by other simple means because the epidemiology is relatively simple.

As stated previously, the single known source of infection is concentrated feedstuffs containing contaminated meat and bone meal. The only major uncertainty is whether there are any natural routes of infection between cattle. By analogy with scrapie, the most likely possibility is transmission of infection from cow to calf. A major experiment has been set up in the United Kingdom to investigate this (see The possibility of endemic infection, p. 55). There are two ways in which countries without BSE might acquire it: first, by the importation of live animals and contaminated feedstuffs from countries with BSE; and second, by allowing endemic scrapie to infect cattle (see Sterilization of meat and bone meal, p. 47, and Restricted use of meat and bone meal, p. 49). Both are easily prevented.

RESTRICTIONS ON TRADE IN LIVE CATTLE

There is obviously a chance that some breeding animals imported from the United Kingdom, for example, might be infected with BSE. Unless large numbers of animals are imported, the statistical probability is quite small. The occurrences of BSE in Oman (Carolan, Wells and Wilesmith, 1990) and the Falkland Islands are the only definite instances of this to date. The long incubation period of BSE means that quarantine is of limited practical value except in special circumstances when the need to import animals outweighs the difficulties and expense of a quarantine period lasting several years.

If there are no natural routes for the spread of infection from cattle to cattle, the only risk from imported livestock would be after slaughter, when infected material might enter the animal feed chain. The chances of this infecting other cattle would be quite small because of extensive dilution with uninfected material. The risk should be zero from animals born in the United Kingdom after the ruminant protein ban came into effect in July 1988.

Nevertheless, natural transmission of BSE infection in cattle is still a possibility (Anon., 1991b). Because of this, the CEC limited the importation of live cattle from the United Kingdom to animals born after July 1988, provided that they were not born to suspect or confirmed BSE cows (CEC,1989).

A later amendment (CEC, 1990a) further restricted imports of live cattle from the United Kingdom to young calves which have to be slaughtered by six months of age in the importing country. This amendment solves the problem of the importing countries having to remove and dispose of the specified bovine offals in line with United Kingdom legislation. The specified offals ban was introduced as a precautionary public health measure but it does not apply to young calves (of six months or less) because no part of these animals is considered to be a significant risk even if they are infected (see Minimizing exposure of the human population, p. 50).

An increasing number of cattle in the United Kingdom have never been fed ruminant protein. Trade in live animals born there after the ruminant protein ban would thus not be a risk to importing countries unless there is cattle-to-cattle transmission of infection. The OIE has recommended specific conditions for the trade in live cattle embryos from countries with high or low incidences of BSE (OIE, 1992).

RESTRICTIONS ON TRADE IN MEAT AND BONE MEAL

The United Kingdom has introduced two restrictions on the use of meat and bone meal in ruminant feeds. The first is a complete ban on the feeding of ruminant-derived protein to ruminants, which was introduced to control BSE by preventing new infections from contaminated feeds (HMSO, 1988a).

The second restriction came in later, initially for public health reasons (see Minimizing exposure of the human population, p. 50) and latterly for animal health reasons (see Minimizing the exposure of other species, p. 53). This bans the use of certain specified bovine offals in human food and animal feedstuffs. The banned offals are those likely to contain the highest amounts of BSE agent in infected cattle. The second restriction also prevents the export to other EEC Member States of specified offals from all bovine animals over the age of six months, and any food products derived from them (HMSO, 1990b).

However, there are no United Kingdom restrictions on the export of meat and bone meal derived from the non-specified bovine wastes (which would have very little infectivity) or material derived from sheep (which would have a significant amount of infectivity). Nor has the EEC imposed any restrictions on trade in meat and bone meal (although several member countries have banned imports from the United Kingdom).

Since the feeding of material of ovine origin to cattle is believed to have been the origin of the BSE epidemic in the United Kingdom, countries wishing to import British meat and bone meal from this country would be well advised not to feed it to ruminants. The feeding of meat and bone meal from other countries with scrapie is considered below.

STERILIZATION OF MEAT AND BONE MEAL

The epidemiology studies described in Chapter 4 show that the potential for BSE to occur in the United Kingdom existed for a long time before the epidemic actually started. One of the lessons of BSE is that a similar potential may exist in other countries.

The occurrence of BSE depends on the simultaneous presence of three factors (Wilesmith and Wells, 1991):

- a large sheep population (in relation to that of cattle) with a sufficient level of endemic scrapie;
- the use of substantial quantities of meat and bone meal derived from sheep, in cattle feed;
- conditions of rendering that allow the survival of significant amounts of infectivity (which will depend on the extent of the initial contamination).

The very low average level of exposure of cattle in the United Kingdom illustrates how nearly the epidemic might have been avoided if any one of these factors had been limiting. The need for all three factors is the reason why few if any other countries in the world are likely to experience BSE on the scale of the United Kingdom epidemic. But there is a real danger of BSE occurring regionally whenever a local combination of these factors leads to the infection of cattle from sheep. Although the reasons for the recent cases of BSE in Switzerland and France are not known, these are the kind of occasional outbreaks to be expected. The United States Department of Agriculture (USDA) has made a detailed analysis of the BSE factors at both national and regional levels (USDA, 1991a; 1991b).

BSE can be prevented by removing any one of the above three factors. In practice, neither the eradication of endemic scrapie nor the depopulation of sheep is a realistic option except in countries which are already close to being in one or other of these positions. Australia and New Zealand are the two major sheep-rearing countries which are generally regarded as scrapie-free. But several others have witnessed little or no scrapie in recent years.

This leaves two major approaches for the prevention of BSE from sheep scrapie. The first is to ensure that meat and bone meal is produced under conditions that achieve total disinfection of the most heat-resistant strains of infectious agent (see below). The second is to avoid the use of meat and bone meal in feedstuffs (see Restricted use of meat and bone meal, p. 49).

For economic reasons, few modern processes still use solvent extraction, which, as previously mentioned, was an important factor in limiting the exposure of cattle in the United Kingdom before 1981/82. With most processes, disinfection of scrapie relies on heating. In common with several other microbial agents, the heat sensitivity of scrapie is greatest in the presence of water. Since most rendering plants operate at atmosphericpressure, the wet-heating stage will take place at temperatures up to about 100 °C, to which the scrapie agent is substantially resistant.

Higher temperatures will be achieved once most of the water has been removed. Wilesmith Ryan and Atkinson (1991) found that the mean temperature achieved in different United Kingdom plants was 124 °C and the maximum was about 150 °C. Undoubtedly, these temperatures would produce some inactivation. The absence of data, however, makes it difficult to ascertain how much infectivity would be lost under different heating conditions (Taylor, 1989a).

In theory, a simple way to inactivate the scrapie/BSE agent is to employ the standard conditions currently used for the disinfection of the CJD agent in United Kingdom hospitals, namely autoclaving at 134-138 °C for 18 minutes (DHSS, 1984). This standard is based on the most heat-stable strain of scrapie (Kimberlin *et al.*, 1983). However, there is a big difference between the porous load sterilization of surgical instruments in hospitals and the steam sterilization of large amounts of either untreated abattoir waste or meat and bone meal (Taylor, 1989a). The practicalities and the effectiveness of such treatments need careful investigation. These studies are in progress but they will take a few years to complete.

RESTRICTED USE OF MEAT AND BONE MEAL

By far the simplest way to prevent BSE is to avoid the use of meat and bone meal, and any other sources of ruminant protein, in cattle feed. This approach can take more than one form.

Material from sheep can be rendered separately from that of other species and specifically excluded from cattle feed. But this would not prevent the recycling of infection that was already present in cattle. This is why the United Kingdom ruminant protein ban applied to material derived from all ruminants, including cattle (HMSO, 1988a).

The ban also applied to the feeding of ruminant protein to sheep (as well as to cattle and deer) to prevent the recycling of scrapie infection in the sheep population which, in the past, may have contributed to endemic scrapie.

The most effective approach is a complete ban on the feeding of all ruminant protein to ruminants, as originally introduced and maintained in the United Kingdom (HMSO, 1988a; 1988e; 1989a; 1990b). This would prevent the feed-borne spread of infection to cattle from both native flocks and imported sheep. It would also prevent the recycling of infection from imported adult United Kingdom cattle which may have been infected, but were too young to show clinical signs of BSE at the time of slaughter.

Such a measure would also take account of the formal possibility that BSE infection may already exist in other countries, quite independently of the United Kingdom and the Republic of Ireland. However unlikely this possibility may seem, the recycling of in apparent infection in cattle could create just the conditions for the selection of more highly neurovirulent strains that could lead to a disease problem.

Several countries, including the United States and members of the EEC, have initiated surveillance programmes to detect evidence of BSE in their national herds. The EEC has made BSE a notifiable disease with effect from 1 April 1990 (CEC, 1990a). The surveillance programmes are based on the histological examination of brain sections from older cattle showing neurological signs. An obvious source of material is suspect cases of rabies. But, until such studies provide evidence to the contrary, it would be prudent to prevent the feed-borne spread of inapparent BSE infection between cattle.

MINIMIZING EXPOSURE OF THE HUMAN POPULATION

A great deal of concern, much of it avoidable, has been expressed over the possible public health consequences of BSE. This is understandable given that the scrapie family of diseases includes some that affect human beings. But the very existence of human scrapie-like diseases long before BSE was discovered means that the possible epidemiological relationships between the animal and human diseases have already been the subject of intensive study. As a result, the circumstances in which BSE might pose a risk to public health can be defined quite precisely, and simple measures have been devised to preempt this risk. This issue was considered in the "Southwood report" (DoH and MAFF, 1989) and it has been discussed at length elsewhere (Kimberlin, 1990b; 1990c; Taylor, 1989b). The salient features of the problem and its solution are described below.

The problem

If scrapie or BSE were to cause disease in human beings, it would probably be recognizable as CJD. Although the epidemiology of CJD is not understood in detail, the possibility that it is caused by scrapie infection of human has been studied and the evidence is firmly against such a causal link. Plausible hypotheses for CJD are discussed elsewhere (Kimberlin, 1990a).

It is highly improbable that the absence of an aetiological link between CJD and scrapie is because human beings have never been exposed to scrapie. On the contrary, their exposure to scrapie infection must have been considerable in several countries for very long periods of time. But, as the epidemiological evidence shows, such exposure has not been high enough to overcome the species barrier which limits the interspecies transmission of these diseases.

In the absence of a demonstrable public health risk from scrapie, the same could well apply to BSE. The only circumstance which could alter this assessment is if the transmission of scrapie to cattle has considerably increased the effective exposure of human beings to infection. The greatest uncertainty would be if cattle had selected scrapie strains which differ from those pre-existing in sheep. That such a possibility exists is demonstrated by laboratory studies of single (cloned) strains of scrapie in mice showing that crossing the species barrier (into hamsters) can permit the selection of mutants with different biological properties from the original strains (Kimberlin, Cole and Walker, 1987; Kimberlin, Walker and Fraser, 1989).

As shown previously, the recycling of BSE infection in the cattle population would have favoured the selection of cattle-adapted strains. Rendering processes may also have had a selective effect by favouring heat-stable strains of agent. However, strain selection per se would not necessarily create a problem because the selected strains could be even less likely than scrapie to cross the species barrier to human beings. The only concern is if they happened to be more able to infect the human population. Unfortunately, there is no easy way of testing this possibility.

It is important to emphasize that any primary human exposure would still be across a species barrier and there would be no recycling of food-borne infection in the human population, as happened with kuru and with BSE in cattle. Nevertheless, there is a theoretical risk to human beings from a disadvantageous selection of BSE strains. The logical way to address this risk is to make sure that exposure to BSE is kept low.

The solution

Attention in the United Kingdom was initially focused on clinically affected cattle which were excluded from the human food chain from August 1988 (HMSO, 1988b). Soon afterwards, the destruction of milk from suspect cases was enforced (HMSO, 1988d; 1988e).

As the number of BSE cases continued to increase, however, there was concern that some animals, at a very early stage of the clinical disease, might escape detection. Even more worrying was the possibility that infected animals were being slaughtered for meat before the age at which clinical signs appear (two years and over). If cattle are dead-end hosts for infection, the number of subclinically infected animals would decrease progressively since the introduction of the meat and bone meal ban in July 1988. But efficient maternal transmission of infection, if it occurred, could change this situation.

This possibility was countered by banning certain specified types of bovine offal from entering the human food chain. The ban came into effect in England and Wales in November 1989 (HMSO, 1989b), and in Scotland and Northern Ireland in January 1990.

The basis of the specified offals ban is that agents in the scrapie family only multiply to an appreciable extent in a small number of tissues (Hadlow, Kennedy and Race, 1982). Indeed, limitations on multiplication and on the cell-to-cell spread of infection are the underlying reason for the long incubation periods of all these diseases (Kimberlin, 1990a).

Most tissues, including milk and muscle, have little or no detectable infectivity by parenteral injection, and effectively none at all by alimentary exposure (because of major differences between routes in the relative efficiency of infection). This is borne out by feeding large quantities of various bovine tissues from BSE cases to mice. Only those mice which were fed brain became infected (Barlow and Middleton, 1990a; 1990b).

There are few bovine tissues used in human food which also have the potential to support significant multiplication of the agent. The most important, quantitatively, are brain, spinal cord, tonsil, spleen, thymus and intestine (the last because of the presence of Peyer's patches). These are the specified offals that are excluded by the ban (HMSO, 1989b).

To be effective, the specified offals ban has had to be applied to all cattle regardless of whether they are infected. The only exception is calves of under six months of age which are exempted on the grounds that none would have been fed ruminant-derived meat and bone meal and, even if there is maternal transmission of infection, little or no detectable infectivity would be expected (from studies of scrapie) in any tissues.

A major feature of the offals ban is that it safeguards public health even if BSE develops into an endemic infection of cattle (see The possibility of endemic infection, p. 55). In other words, it separates the animal health and the public health aspects of BSE.

Logically, the ban should also be applied to the large lymphnodes. In the United Kingdom, these are removed as a matter of course,along with other waste tissue (including large nerves), either in the abattoir or when individual cuts of meat are prepared. In 1990 these steps were given added force by EEC decisions taken to facilitate trade in United Kingdom beef.

For boneless beef, there is a requirement to remove obvious nervous and lymphatic tissue during the cutting process before export (CEC, 1990b). These trimmings are excluded from use in human food. For bone-in beef, the animals must not come from a holding in which BSE has been confirmed in the previous two years (CEC, 1990b). The scientific basis for this second measure is dubious but it was expedient for political reasons.

The OIE initially endorsed these conditions for the trade in meat and meat products for human consumption from countries with a high incidence of BSE (OIE, 1990). Subsequently, the organization recommended that the conditions for trade in bone-in beef should be the same as for boneless beef (OIE, 1992). The OIE has also recommended that there are no grounds for restrictions in trade in milk or milk products because of BSE (OIE, 1990; 1992).

MINIMIZING THE EXPOSURE OF OTHER SPECIES

During the time that cattle were exposed to contaminated meat and bone meal, which led to BSE, pigs were also exposed with no ill effects. Indeed, the exposure of pigs would have been higher than cattle because of the greater inclusion rates of meat and bone meal in commercial pig feeds.

If the effective exposure had been the same for both species, about 1 000 cases of spongiform encephalopathy would have been seen by now in the population of breeding sows in the United Kingdom. The clinical appearance of porcine spongiform encephalopathy is known from studies of the experimental disease (Dawson, Wells, Parker and Scott, 1990), and it is improbable that a naturally occurring disease in pigs would have been undetected. It must be concluded that an effective exposure to produce the disease in cattle was insufficient in pigs.

The ruminant protein ban, introduced in 1988 to control BSE, did not apply to pigs, which have continued to be exposed along with some other species. Two events in 1990 led to a reappraisal of the risks to pigs and other species.

First, the scale of the recycling of infection within the cattle population and its effect on the BSE epidemic became clear. As shown in Chapter 4, the consequences of recycling include changes not only in the amount of infectivity but, possibly, in the strains of agent. In other words, it could not be assumed that the effective exposure of pigs would stay constant.

The second event was the occurrence of several cases of spongiform encephalopathy in domestic cats (Wyatt *et al.*, 1990; Leggett, Dukes and Pirie, 1990). It is too early to know the reasons for the feline cases, but it may be significant that they have occurred relatively late in the BSE epidemic. One possibility is that feline spongiform encephalopathy may have been a consequence of changes in the character (strain and effective dose) of BSE infection of cattle.

For these two reasons, it was desirable on animal health grounds to reduce the exposure of all animal species to BSE. The introduction of the specified offals ban in 1989 made this easy to achieve without a complete ban on the use of all meat and bone meal in feeds. Because the specified offals include the major tissues likely to contain high BSE infectivity, all that was needed was to extend the specified offals ban. Since September 1990 these bovine offals may not be fed in any form to any species of mammal or bird (HMSO, 1990b).

Chapter 9
Control and eradication

There are two scenarios for the future course of BSE. The first is that BSE, like TME and kuru, is a dead-end disease. If this is true, and if meat and bone meal was the sole source of the infection, then removing this source would be sufficient for the eventual eradication of BSE from the United Kingdom.

In July 1988, the United Kingdom Government introduced a ban on the feeding of all ruminant-derived protein to ruminants (HMSO, 1988a; for subsequent modifications see HMSO, 1988e; 1989a; 1990b). However, the incubation period of BSE in cattle averages about four to five years. This means that no reduction in the current incidence can be expected until 1992 at the earliest.

THE POSSIBILITY OF ENDEMIC INFECTION

The alternative scenario is that there are natural routes of transmission of BSE and that the outbreak could turn into an endemic infection of cattle in the way that scrapie is in sheep.

As of July 1991 the ongoing epidemiological survey had not revealed any firm evidence of maternal transmission of BSE, as would be expected from the analogy with scrapie. Only one putative case of maternal transmission in cattle has been reported (Anon., 1991b).

A major experiment was set up in 1989 in order to investigate this question. Carefully matched groups of test and control animals are being observed to see if the incidence of BSE is higher in calves born to BSE-affected dams. A high level of maternal transmission of infection could be manifest after 1992. A much longer observation period (up to a maximum of seven years) will be necessary to prove a low incidence of maternal transmission or to show that it does not occur.

To sustain BSE infection in the cattle population requires that each breeding cow is replaced by at least one infected female calf, which then transmits infection to at least one of her offspring. The current breeding regimes in the United Kingdom dairy herds, with an annual herd replacement rate of 20 to 25 percent, would not enable this to occur for a prolonged period of time, even with a 100 percent maternal transmission of infection to calves. Therefore, the worst that could happen in this situation is that the rate of decline in the incidence of BSE would be somewhat slower than if BSE were a dead-end infection (Wilesmith and Wells, 1991).

For BSE to become endemic, the number of infected cattle would need to increase by horizontal spread. In scrapie, this can occur particularly at lambing as a by-product of the postnatal component of maternal transmission. For example, an infected placenta can be a source of infection to unrelated ewes.

Cattle management is sufficiently different from sheep management for the chances of horizontal spread of BSE to be lower, especially in dairy herds where cows often calve in isolation and the calves are separated after a few days.

The same is not true of beef suckler herds in which cows and calves run together. This would increase the chances of postnatal maternal transmission and it might also create opportunities for the horizontal spread of infection. However, BSE is much rarer in beef than in dairy herds (see Table 4 and Wilesmith *et al.*, 1988; 1992a).

In conclusion, BSE is unlikely to become an endemic infection of cattle unless a high level of maternal transmission enables the epidemic to be amplified by the horizontal spread of infection. It is too soon to assess this possibility but it seems improbable that BSE is highly contagious because the average incidence within affected herds is only about 2 percent. There is little point in imposing additional control measures until there is a demonstrable need for them. However, common sense urges two simple precautionary steps. The first is that calves born to cows which are or which become confirmed cases of BSE should not be selected as replacement heifers within the herd. The existence in the United Kingdom of a specified offals ban means that such calves could, for example, be fattened for beef without risk to public health.

The second recommendation is to minimize the risk of horizontal spread of infection at calving by good hygiene and the early disposal of the placenta (by incineration or burial). This is a legal requirement on those rare occasions when a suspect BSE case is calving (HMSO, 1988b), but it is good practice for reducing the spread of other infections as well.

THE WORST-CASE SCENARIO

Although unlikely, the worst possible situation would be if BSE became established as an endemic infection in exactly the same manner as scrapie. The difficulties of eradication would then be similar.

Scrapie can be controlled quite effectively by selective culling in the female line and by husbandry measures to limit the horizontal spread of infection at lambing. But two problems make this a difficult task.

The first is the need for accurate breeding records, which rarely exist when most needed, at the start of the outbreak. Selective culling cannot begin without them and it takes several years to build up sufficient records.

The second problem is that infected ewe lines can only be identified when the clinical disease appears. The spread of infection from a ewe to several successive lamb crops can easily go unnoticed for a generation if the animal dies or is culled before developing the clinical disease. Since only a small proportion of ewe lambs may be retained for breeding, another infected generation could be missed if the few lambs that survive as breeding ewes happen to be of a sip genotype which can be infected but never develops the disease.

It therefore requires many years of patient application to bring scrapie under control. Much of the work can easily be undone if bought-in flock replacements reintroduce the infection. This is why the eradication of scrapie is so difficult. The same problems could attend the eradication of BSE, with one important difference, described below.

In sheep, the sip gene has a major effect in controlling the susceptibility and incubation period of scrapie. Sip and PrP genes in sheep are almost certainly the same. The PrP gene is also present in cattle, and allelic variants have been found which have either five or six copies of an octapeptide repeat sequence in the coding region (Goldmann *et al.*, 1991).

However, studies of a large herd affected with multiple cases showed no association of BSE with this polymorphism of the PrP gene (Dawson and Martin, personal communication). These findings are consistent with the biological evidence (particularly from transmission studies as mentioned in Chapter 4, suggesting that there may be little or no allelic variation at the PrP or any other genetic locus that affects BSE. If true, the occurrence of infected carriers may be far less common in BSE than in scrapie, making BSE easier to eradicate.

If further steps to eradicate BSE become necessary, they would not be worth applying on less than a national scale. The essential prerequisite is good breeding and movement records which are currently being compiled in the United Kingdom following recent legislation (HMSO, 1990c; 1990d). By the time they are sufficient for the task, the necessity (or otherwise) for further action to eradicate BSE will be known. Meanwhile, the precautionary measures to safeguard other species, including human beings, are already in place.

Appendix

Protocol for the histopathological diagnosis of bovine spongiform encephalopathy

PRIMARY FIXATION

The fixative, 10 percent formol saline, is prepared by dissolving 8.5 g of sodium chloride in 900 ml of distilled water and mixing with 100 ml of 40 percent formaldehyde. The whole uncut brain is fixed in 10 percent formol saline using 10 to 20 times the volume of brain, i.e. 4 to 8 litres of fixative. Change the fixative after one week and retain for a further week. If necessary, the brain can be transported in a smaller volume of fixative to a diagnostic centre with appropriate packaging to ensure it safe transit (see Barlow, 1983).

CUTTING IN

The brain should be cut coronally at 3 to 5 mm intervals. Four brain stem blocks are selected for processing. The recommended sites are: the medulla, at the obex; the medulla, through the rostral cerebellar peduncles; the midbrain, at two levels to include the superior colliculus and the red nucleus.

SECONDARY FIXATION

The selected blocks are returned to fresh formol saline for a further week during which time the fixative should be changed three times before processing. Mechanical agitation of the blocks (e.g. with an orbital shaker) enhances penetration of the fixative.

HISTOLOGICAL PROCESSING

Tissues should be rinsed in 70 percent alcohol before being placed on the processor. The schedule for a carousel-type processor is shown in Box 1.

Box 1. Schedule for a carousel-type processor

70% alcohol	2 x 30 minutes
90% alcohol	2 x 30 minutes
100% alcohol	3 x 1 hour
Chloroform I	1 x 1 hour
Chloroform II	14 hours
Wax I	2 hours
Wax II	1 hour
Wax III	1 hour

Notes:
i) The time in chloroform should be adjusted to the maximum that the processor will accommodate within the range of 12 to 18 hours.
ii) Reagents should be changed frequently - after three runs would be a guideline.

STAINING

The staining schedule for haematoxylin and eosin is shown in Box 2.

HISTOPATHOLOGICAL EXAMINATION

Bright field, light microscopic examination is carried out according to standard histopathological practice.

DIAGNOSTIC CRITERIA

The following guidelines for diagnostic criteria should apply:

- *Positive*. The presence of vacuolation affecting grey matter neuropil and neuronal perikarya with a systematic and usually bilaterally symmetrical distribution (see Wells *et al.*, 1987).

  Note that neuronal vacuolation in the red nucleus is an incidental finding in cattle brains and its occurrence must be disregarded for the purpose of BSE diagnosis.

Box 2. Staining schedule for haematoxylin and eosin

De-wax sections in xylene	2 x 2 minutes
Absolute alcohol	2 x 1 minute
70% alcohol	30 seconds
Tap-water	2 minutes
Harris' haematoxylin - acidified	8 minutes*
Rinse in tap.water	2 minutes
Acid alcohol (0.1% hydrochloric acid)	10 seconds
Wash in tap-water	5 minutes
"Blue" in saturated (1.5%) lithiumcarbonate	30 seconds
Wash in tap-water	10 minutes
Eosin ("yellowish" - 2% in tap water-plus formalin to 0.2%)	4 minutes
Running water	5 minutes
Absolute alcohol	2 x 2 minutes
Xylene	3 x 1 minute
Mount in DPX	

* The time in haematoxylin will need to be adjusted to provide the correct intensity of stain.

Notes:
i) Where necessary, use "Scotts Tap-water Substitute" instead of tap-water.
ii) Acidified Harris' Haematoxylin: CLIN-Tech, 1-2 Faraday Way, London SE18 5TR.
iii) EOSIN. Yellowish. C. 1 45380, BDH/MERCK.

• *Inconclusive.*

i) Inadequate submission of material with poor representation of lesion target sites or severe postmortem change;

ii) vacuolation of the grey matter neuropil and/or neuronal perikarya evident only as a minimal change.

Note that in all cases where the initial examination is inconclusive, further tissue sampling, processing and examination should be undertaken at the pathologist's discretion.

- *Negative.*

  i) Absence of lesions in a range of sections which adequately represent lesion target sites;

  ii) lesions indicating an alternative neuropathological diagnosis with absence of vacuolar changes in BSE lesion target sites.

  Note that where clinical signs have strongly suggested BSE, or an alternative diagnosis, further sampling should be undertaken at the pathologist's discretion to reach a diagnosis.
- *Unresolved.* In a few cases, the pathologist may be undecided and/or unable to classify the histopathology, and may wish to have a second opinion before classifying into one of the other three categories.

References

Aldridge, B.M., Scott, P.R., Holmes, L.A., Milne, E.M. & Collins, D.F. 1988. Elevated plasma glucose concentration in a case of bovine spongiform encephalopathy. *Vet. Rec.*, 122: 71-72.

Anon. 1990a. BSE case found on the continent. *Vet. Rec.*, 127: 462.

Anon. 1990b. Spongiform encephalopathy confirmed in a young kudu. *Vet. Rec.*, 127: 606.

Anon. 1991a. BSE case confirmed in Brittany. *Vet. Rec.*, 128: 218.

Anon. 1991b. BSE found in calf born after start of feed ban. *Vet. Rec.*, 128: 314.

Barlow, R.M. 1983. Neurological disorders of cattle and sheep. *Practice*, 5: 77.

Barlow, R.M. & Middleton, D.J. 1990a. Dietary transmission of bovine spongiform encephalopathy to mice. *Vet. Rec.*, 126: 111-112.

Barlow, R.M. & Middleton, D.J. 1990b. Is BSE simply scrapie in cattle? *Vet. Rec.*, 126: 295.

Basset, H. & Sheridan, C. 1989. Case of BSE in the Irish Republic. *Vet. Rec.*, 124: 151.

Carolan, D.J.P., Wells, G.A.H. & Wilesmith, J.W. 1990. BSE in Oman. *Vet. Rec.*, 126: 92.

CEC. 1989. *Commission of the European Communities Decision 89/469*, 28 July 1989.

CEC. 1990a. *Commission of the European Communities Decision 90/134*, 6 March 1990.

CEC. 1990b. *Commission of the European Communities Decision 90/261*, 8 June 1990.

Cranwell, M.P., Hancock, R.D., Hindson, J.R., Hall, S.A., Daniel, N.J., Hopkins, A.R., Wonnacott, B., Vivian, M. & Hunt, P. 1988. Bovine spongiform encephalopathy. *Vet. Rec.*, 122: 190.

Dawson, M., Wells, G.A.H. & Parker, B.N.J. 1990. Preliminary evidence of the experimental transmissibility of bovine spongiform encephalopathy to cattle. *Vet. Rec.*, 126: 112-113.

Dawson, M., Wells, G.A.H., Parker, B.N.J. & Scott, A.C. 1990. Primary parenteral transmission of bovine spongiform encephalopathy to the pig. *Vet. Rec.*, 127: 338.

Dawson, M., Wells, G.A.H., Parker,

B.N.J. & Scott, A.C. 1991. Transmission studies of BSE in cattle, hamsters, pigs and domestic fowl. *In* R. Bradley, M. Savey & B.A. Marchant, eds. *Sub-acute Spongiform Encephalopathies. Current Topics in Veterinary Medicine and Animal Science,* 55: 25-32. Dordrecht, the Netherlands, Kluwer Academic Press.

Denny, G.O., Wilesmith, J.W., Clements, R.A. & Hueston, W.D. 1991. Bovine spongiform encephalopathy in Northern Ireland: epidemiological observations 1988-1990. *Vet. Rec.*, 130: 113-116.

DHSS. 1984. *The Management of Patients with Spongiform Encephalopathy (Creutzfeldt-Jakob Disease).* Department of Health and Social Security Circular DA (84) 16.

DoH and MAFF. 1989. *Report of the Working Party on Bovine Spongiform Encephalopathy.* London, Department of Health.

Fleetwood, A.J. & Furley, C.W. 1990. Spongiform encephalopathy in an eland. *Vet. Rec.*, 126: 408-409.

Fraser, H., Bruce, M.E. & McConnell, I. 1991. Murine scrapie strains, BSE models and genetics. *In* R. Bradley, M. Savey & B.A. Marchant, eds. *Sub-acute Spongiform Encephalopathies. Current Topics in Veterinary Medicine and Animal Science,* 55: 131-136. Dordrecht, the Netherlands, Kluwer Academic Press.

Fraser, H., McConnell, I., Wells, G.A.H. & Dawson, M. 1988. Transmission of bovine spongiform encephalopathy to mice. *Vet. Rec.*, 123: 472.

Gibbs, C.J. Jr, Safar, J., Ceroni, M., Di Martino, A., Clark, W.W. & Hourrigan, J.L. 1990. Experimental transmission of scrapie to cattle. *The Lancet,* 335: 1275.

Gilmour, J.S., Buxton, D., Macleod, N.S.M., Brodie, T.A. & More, J.B. 1988. Bovine spongiform encephalopathy. *Vet. Rec.*, 122: 142.

Goldmann, W., Hunter, N., Martin, T., Dawson, M. & Hope, J. 1991. Different forms of the bovine PrP gene have five or six copies of a short, G-C-rich element within the protein-coding exon. *J. Gen. Virol.*, 72: 201-204.

Hadlow, W.J., Kennedy, R.C. & Race, R.E. 1982. Natural infection of Suffolk sheep with scrapie virus. *J. Infect. Dis.,* 146: 657.

HMSO. 1985. *Animal waste. A report on the supply of animal waste in Great Britain.* London, Monopolies and Mergers Commission.

HMSO. 1988a. *The Bovine Spongiform Encephalopathy Order 1988.* Statutory Instrument 1988, no. 1039. London.

HMSO. 1988b. *The Bovine Spongiform Encephalopathy (Amendment) Order 1988*. Statutory Instrument 1988, no. 1345. London.

HMSO. 1988c. *The Bovine Spongiform Encephalopathy Compensation Order 1988*. Statutory Instrument 1988, no. 1346. London.

HMSO. 1988d. *The Zoonoses Order 1988*. Statutory Instrument 1988, no. 2264. London.

HMSO. 1988e. *The Bovine Spongiform Encephalopathy (no. 2) Order 1988.* Statutory Instrument 1988, no. 2299. London.

HMSO. 1989a. *The Bovine Spongiform Encephalopathy (no. 2) Amendment Order 1989*. Statutory Instrument 1989, no. 2326. London.

HMSO. 1989b. *The Bovine Offal (Prohibition) Regulations 1989*. Statutory Instrument 1989 no. 2061.

HMSO. 1990a. *The Bovine Spongiform Encephalopathy Compensation Order 1990*. Statutory Instrument 1990, no. 222. London.

HMSO. 1990b. *The Bovine Spongiform Encephalopathy (no. 2) Amendment Order 1990*. Statutory Instrument 1990, no. 1930. London.

HMSO. 1990c. *The Bovine Animals (Identification, Marking and Breeding Records) Order 1990*. Statutory Instrument 1990, no. 1867. London.

HMSO. 1990d. *The Movement of Animals (Records) (Amendment) Order 1990*. Statutory Instrument 1990, no. 1868. London.

Hope, J., Reekie, L.J.D., Hunter, N., Multhaup, G., Beyreuther, K., White, H., Scott, A.C., Stack, M.J., Dawson, M. & Wells, G.A.H. 1988. Fibrils from brains of cows with new cattle disease contain scrapie-associated protein. *Nature (London)*, 336: 390-392.

Jeffrey, M. & Wells, G.A.H. 1988. Spongiform encephalopathyin a nyala *(Tragelaphus angasi)*. *Vet. Path.* 25: 398-399.

Johnson, C.T. & Whitaker, C.J. 1988. Bovine spongiform encephalopathy. *Vet. Rec.*, 122: 142.

Kimberlin, R.H. 1990a. Unconventional "slow" viruses. *In* L.H. Collier & M.C. Timbury, eds. *Topley and Wilson's principles of bacteriology, virology and immunity.* 8th ed, vol. 4, p. 671-693. London, Edward Arnold.

Kimberlin, R.H. 1990b. Bovine spongiform encephalopathy. *In* L.K. Borysiewicz, ed. *Horizons in medicine,* no. 2, p. 274-283. Tunbridge Wells, Kent, Transmedica Europe Limited.

Kimberlin, R.H. 1990c. Bovine spongiform encephalopathy: taking stock of the issues. *Nature (London),* 345: 763-764.

Kimberlin, R.H., Cole, S. & Walker, C.A. 1987. Temporary and permanent modifications to a single strain of mouse scrapie on transmission to rats and hamsters. *J. Gen. Virol.*, 68: 1875-1881.

Kimberlin, R.H., Walker, C.A. & Fraser, H. 1989. The genomic identity of different strains of mouse scrapie is expressed in hamsters and preserved on reisolation in mice. *J. Gen. Virol.*, 70: 2017-2025.

Kimberlin, R.H., Walker, C.A., Millson, G.C., Taylor, D.M., Robertson, P.A., Tomlinson, A.H. & Dickinson, A.G. 1983. Disinfection studies with two strains of mouse-passaged scrapie agent. *J. Neurol. Sci.*, 59: 355-369.

Kirkwood, J.K., Wells, G.A.H., Wilesmith, J.W., Cunningham, A.A. & Jackson, S.I. 1990. Spongiform encephalopathy in an arabian oryx *(Oryx leucoryx)* and a greater kudu *(Tragelaphus strepsiceros)*. *Vet. Rec.*, 127: 418-420.

Kirkwood, J.K., Wells, G.A.H., Cunningham, A.A., Jackson, S.I., Scott, A.C., Dawson, M. & Wilesmith, J.W. 1992. Scrapie-like encephalopathy in greater kudu *(Tragelaphus strepsiceros)*: morbidity in an index case offspring without dietary exposure to ruminant-derived protein. *Vet. Rec.*, 130.

Leggett, M.M., Dukes, J. & Pirie, H.M. 1990. A spongiform encephalopathy in a cat. *Vet. Rec.*, 127: 586-588.

Liberski, P.P. 1990. Ultrastructural neuropathologic features of bovine spongiform encephalopathy. *J. Am. Vet. Med. Assoc.*, 196: 1682.

Marsh, R.F., Bessen, R.A., Lehmann, S. & Hartsough, G.R. 1991. Epidemiological and experimental studies on a new incident of transmissible mink encephalopathy. *J. Gen. Virol.*, 72: 589-594.

Matthews, D. 1990. Bovine spongiform encephalopathy (BSE) – the story so far. *State Vet. J.* 44: 3-18.

OIE. 1990. *Recommendation No. 2.* Adopted 5 October 1990 by the 14th Conference of the Office international des epizooties Regional Commission for Europe, Sofia, Bulgaria.

OIE. 1992. *International Animal Health Code.* Chapter 3.2.13.

Scott, P.R., Aldridge, B.M., Holmes, L.A., Milne, E.M. & Collins, D.M. 1988. Bovine spongiform encephalopathy in an adult British Friesian cow. *Vet. Rec.*, 123: 373-374.

Scott, P.R., Aldridge, B.M., Clarke, M. & Will, R. 1989. Bovine spongiform encephalopathy in a cow in the United Kingdom. *J. Am. Vet. Med. Assoc.*, 195: 1745-1747.

Scott, P.R., Aldridge, B.M., Clarke, M. & Will, R. 1990a. Cerebrospinal fluid studies in normal cows and cases of bovine spongiform encephalopathy. *Br. Vet. J.*, 146: 88-90.

Scott, A.C., Wells, G.A.H., Stack, M.J., White, H. & Dawson, M. 1990b. Bovine spongiform encephalopathy: detection and quantitation of fibrils, fibril protein (PrP) and vacuolation in brain. *Vet. Microbiol.*, 23: 295-304.

Taylor, D.M. 1989a. Scrapie agent decontamination: implications for bovine spongiform encephalopathy. *Vet. Rec.*, 24: 291-292.

Taylor, D.M. 1989b. Bovine spongiform encephalopathy and human health. *Vet. Rec.*, 125: 413-415.

USDA. 1991a. *Qualitative analysis of BSE risk factors in the United States.* United States Department of Agriculture, APHIS:VS, Animal Health Information, Fort Collins, Colorado, USA.

USDA. 1991b. *Quantitative risk assessment of BSE in the United States.* United States Department of Agriculture, APHIS:VS, Animal Health Information, Fort Collins, Colo., US.

Wells, G.A.H., Scott, A.C., Johnson, C.T., Gunning, R.F., Hancock, R.D., Jeffrey, M., Dawson, M. & Bradley, R. 1987. A novel progressive spongiform encephalopathy in cattle. *Vet. Rec.*, 121: 419-420.

Wells, G.A.H. & Wells, M. 1989. Neuropil vacuolation in brain: a reproducible histological processing artefact. *J. Comp. Pathol.*, 101: 355-362.

Wells, G.A.H., Hancock, R.D., Cooley, W.A., Richards, M.S., Higgins, R.J. & David, G.P. 1989. Bovine spongiform encephalopathy: diagnostic significance of vacuolar changes in selected nuclei of the medulla oblongata. *Vet. Rec.*, 125: 521-524.

Wells, G.A.H., Wilesmith, J.W. & McGill, I.S. 1991. Bovine spongiform encephalopathy: a neuropathological perspective. *Brain Pathol.* 1: 69-78.

Wijeratne, W.V.S. & Curnow, R.N. 1990. A study of the inheritance of susceptibility to bovine spongiform encephalopathy. *Vet. Rec.*, 126: 5-8.

Wilesmith, J.W. 1991. The epidemiology of bovine spongiform encephalopathy. *Seminars in Virol.* 2: 239-245.

Wilesmith, J.W. 1992. Bovine spongiform encephalopathy: epidemiological approaches, trial and tribulations. In: *Proceedings of the* *sixth international symposium on veterinary epidemiology and economics.*

Wilesmith, J.W., Wells, G.A.H., Cranwell, M.P. & Ryan, J.M.B. 1988. Bovine spongiform encephalopathy: epidemiological studies. *Vet. Rec.*, 123: 638-644.

Wilesmith, J.W., Ryan, J.B.M. & Atkinson, M.J. 1991. Bovine spongiform encephalopathy: epidemiological studies on the origin. *Vet. Rec.*, 128: 199-203.

Wilesmith, J.W. & Wells, G.A.H. 1991. Bovine spongiform encephalopathy. *In* B.W. Chesebro & M. Oldstone, eds. *Transmissible Spongiform Encephalopathies. Current Topics in Microbiology and Immunology*, 172: 21-38. New York, Springer-Verlag.

Wilesmith, J.W., Ryan, J.B.M., Hueston, W.D. & Hoinville, L.J. 1992a. Bovine spongiform encephalopathy: epidemiological features 1985-1990. *Vet. Rec.*, 130: 90-94.

Wilesmith, J.W., Hoinville, L.J., Ryan, J.B.M. & Sayers, A.R. 1992b. Bovine spongiform encephalopathy: aspects of the clinical picture and analyses of possible changes 1986-1990. *Vet. Rec.*, 130: 197-201.

Wilesmith, J.W., Ryan, J.B.M. & Hueston, W.D. 1992c. Bovine spongiform encephalopathy: case-control studies of calf feeding practices and meat and bone meal inclusion in proprietary concentrates. *Research in Veterinary science.*

Williams, E.S., Thorne, E.T., Miller, M., Spraker, T.R. & Neil, P. 1990. Epizootiology of cervid spongiform encephalopathy (chronic wasting disease). *Abstracts of the VIth International Conference on Wildlife Diseases*, p.63. Berlin, Germany.

Winter, M.H., Aldridge, B.M., Scott, P.R. & Clarke, M. 1989. Occurrence of 14 cases of bovine spongiform encephalopathy in a closed dairy herd. *Br. Vet. J.* 145: 191-194.

Wyatt, J.M., Pearson, G.R., Smerdon, T., Gruffydd-Jones, T.J. & Wells, G.A.H. 1990. Spongiform encephalopathy in a cat. *Vet. Rec.*, 126: 513.

Wyatt, J.M., Pearson, G.R., Smerdon, T.N., Gruffydd-Jones, T.J., Wells, G.A.H. & Wilesmith, J.W. 1991. Naturally occurring scrapie-like spongiform encephalopathy in five domestic cats. *Vet. Rec.*, 129: 233-236.

FAO TECHNICAL PAPERS

FAO ANIMAL PRODUCTION AND HEALTH PAPERS

1 Animal breeding: selected articles from the *World Animal Review*, 1977 (C E F S)
2 Eradication of hog cholera and African swine fever, 1976 (E F S)
3 Insecticides and application equipment for tsetse control, 1977 (E F)
4 New feed resources, 1977 (E/F/S)
5 Bibliography of the criollo cattle of the Americas, 1977 (E/S)
6 Mediterranean cattle and sheep in crossbreeding, 1977 (E F)
7 The environmental impact of tsetse control operations, 1977 (E F)
7 Rev. 1. The environmental impact of tsetse control operations, 1980 (E F)
8 Declining breeds of Mediterranean sheep, 1978 (E F)
9 Slaughterhouse and slaughterslab design and construction, 1978 (E F S)
10 Treating straw for animal feeding, 1978 (C E F S)
11 Packaging, storage and distribution of processed milk, 1978 (E)
12 Ruminant nutrition: selected articles from the *World Animal Review*, 1978 (C E F S)
13 Buffalo reproduction and artificial insemination, 1979 (E*)
14 The African trypanosomiases, 1979 (E F)
15 Establishment of dairy training centres, 1979 (E)
16 Open yard housing for young cattle, 1981 (Ar E F S)
17 Prolific tropical sheep, 1980 (E F S)
18 Feed from animal wastes: state of knowledge, 1980 (C E)
19 East Coast fever and related tick-borne diseases, 1980 (E)
20/1 Trypanottolerant livestock in West and Central Africa – Vol. 1. General study, 1980 (E F)
20/2 Trypanotolerant livestock in West and Central Africa – Vol. 2. Country studies, 1980 (E F)
20/3 Le bétail trypanotolérant en Afrique occidentale et centrale – Vol. 3. Bilan d'une décennie, 1988 (F)
21 Guideline for dairy accounting, 1980 (E)
22 Recursos genéticos animales en América Latina, 1981 (S)
23 Disease control in semen and embryos, 1981 (C E F S)
24 Animal genetic resources – conservation and management, 1981 (C E)
25 Reproductive efficiency in cattle, 1982 (C E F S)
26 Camels and camel milk, 1982 (E)
27 Deer farming, 1982 (E)
28 Feed from animal wastes: feeding manual, 1982 (C E)
29 Echinococcosis/hydatidosis surveillance, prevention and control: FAO/UNEP/WHO guidelines, 1982 (E)
30 Sheep and goat breeds of India, 1982 (E)
31 Hormones in animal production, 1982 (E)
32 Crop residues and agro-industrial by-products in animal feeding, 1982 (E/F)
33 Haemorrhagic septicaemia, 1982 (E F)
34 Breeding plans for ruminant livestock in the tropics, 1982 (E F S)
35 Off-tastes in raw and reconstituted milk, 1983 (Ar E F S)
36 Ticks and tick-borne diseases: selected articles from the *World Animal Review*, 1983 (E F S)
37 African animal trypanosomiasis: selected articles from the *World Animal Review*, 1983 (E F)
38 Diagnosis and vaccination for the control of brucellosis in the Near East, 1982 (Ar E)
39 Solar energy in small-scale milk collection and processing, 1983 (E F)
40 Intensive sheep production in the Near East, 1983 (Ar E)
41 Integrating crops and livestock in West Africa, 1983 (E F)
42 Animal energy in agriculture in Africa and Asia, 1984 (E/F S)
43 Olive by-products for animal feed, 1985 (Ar E F S)
44/1 Animal genetic resources conservation by management, data banks and training, 1984 (E)
44/2 Animal genetic resources: cryogenic storage of germplasm and molecular engineering, 1984 (E)
45 Maintenance systems for the dairy plant, 1984 (E)
46 Livestock breeds of China, 1984 (E F S)
47 Réfrigération du lait à la ferme et organisation des transports, 1985 (F)
48 La fromagerie et les variétés de fromages du bassin méditerranéen, 1985 (F)
49 Manual for the slaughter of small ruminants in developing countries, 1985 (E)
50 Better utilization of crop residues and by-products in animal feeding: research guidelines – 1. State of knowledge, 1985 (E)
50/2 Better utilization of crop residues and by-products in animal feeding: research guidelines – 2. A practical manual for research workers, 1986 (E)
51 Dried salted meats: charque and carne-de-sol, 1985 (E)
52 Small-scale sausage production, 1985 (E)
53 Slaughterhouse cleaning and sanitation, 1985 (E)
54 Small ruminants in the Near East – Vol. I. Selected papers presented for the Expert Consultation on Small Ruminant Research and Development in the Near East (Tunis, 1985), 1987 (E)
55 Small ruminants in the Near East – Vol. II. Selected articles from *World Animal Review* 1972-1986, 1987 (Ar E)
56 Sheep and goats in Pakistan, 1985 (E)
57 The Awassi sheep with special reference to the improved dairy type, 1985 (E)
58 Small ruminant production in the developing countries, 1986 (E)
59/1 Animal genetic resources data banks – 1. Computer systems study for regional data banks, 1986 (E)
59/2 Animal genetic resources data banks – 2. Descriptor lists for cattle, buffalo, pigs, sheep and goats, 1986 (E F S)
59/3 Animal genetic resources data banks – 3. Descriptor lists for poultry, 1986 (E F S)
60 Sheep and goats in Turkey, 1986 (E)
61 The Przewalski horse and restoration to its natural habitat in Mongolia, 1986 (E)
62 Milk and dairy products: production and processing costs, 1988 (E F S)
63 Proceedings of the FAO expert consultation on the substitution of imported concentrate feeds in animal production systems in developing countries, 1987 (C E)
64 Poultry management and diseases in the Near East, 1987 (Ar)
65 Animal genetic resources of the USSR, 1989 (E)

66 Animal genetic resources – strategies for improved use and conservation, 1987 (E)
67/1 Trypanotolerant cattle and livestock development in West and Central Africa – Vol. I, 1987 (E)
67/2 Trypanotolerant cattle and livestock development in West and Central Africa – Vol. II, 1987 (E)
68 Crossbreeding *Bos indicus* and *Bos taurus* for milk production in the tropics, 1987 (E)
69 Village milk processing, 1988 (E F S)
70 Sheep and goat meat production in the humid tropics of West Africa, 1989 (E/F)
71 The development of village-based sheep production in West Africa, 1988 (Ar E F S) (Published as Training manual for extension workers, M/S5840E)
72 Sugarcane as feed, 1988 (E/S)
73 Standard design for small-scale modular slaughterhouses, 1988 (E)
74 Small ruminants in the Near East – Vol. III. North Africa, 1989 (E)
75 The eradication of ticks, 1989 (E/S)
76 *Ex situ* cryoconservation of genomes and genes of endangered cattle breeds by means of modern biotechnological methods, 1989 (E)
77 Training manual for embryo transfer in cattle, 1991 (E)
78 Milking, milk production hygiene and udder health, 1989 (E)
79 Manual of simple methods of meat preservation, 1990 (E)
80 Animal genetic resources – a global programme for sustainable development, 1990 (E)
81 Veterinary diagnostic bacteriology – a manual of laboratory procedures of selected diseases of livestock, 1990 (E F)
82 Reproduction in camels – a review, 1990 (E)
83 Training manual on artificial insemination in sheep and goats, 1991 (E)
84 Training manual for embryo transfer in water buffaloes, 1991 (E)
85 The technology of traditional milk products in developing countries, 1990 (E)
86 Feeding dairy cows in the tropics, 1991 (E)
87 Manual for the production of anthrax and blackleg vaccines, 1991 (E F)
88 Small ruminant production and the small ruminant genetic resource in tropical Africa, 1991 (E)
89 Manual for the production of Marek's disease, Gumboro disease and inactivated Newcastle disease vaccines, 1991 (E F)
90 Application of biotechnology to nutrition of animals in developing countries, 1991 (E F)
91 Guidelines for slaughtering, meat cutting and further processing, 1991 (E)
92 Manual on meat cold store operation and management, 1991 (E S)
93 Utilization of renewable energy sources and energy-saving technologies by small-scale milk plants and collection centres, 1992 (E)
94 Proceedings of the FAO expert consultation on the genetic aspects of trypanotolerance, 1992 (E)
95 Roots, tubers, plantains and bananas in animal feeding, 1992 (E)
96 Distribution and impact of helminth diseases of livestock in developing countries, 1992 (E)
97 Construction and operation of medium-sized abattoirs in developing countries, 1992 (E)
98 Small-scale poultry processing, 1992 (E)
99 *In situ* conservation of livestock and poultry, 1992 (E)
100 Programme for the control of African animal trypanosomiasis and related development, 1992 (E)
101 Genetic improvement of hair sheep in the tropics, 1992 (E)
102 Legume trees and other fodder trees as protein sources for livestock, 1992 (E)
103 Improving sheep reproduction in the Near East, 1992 (Ar)
104 The management of global animal genetic resources, 1992 (E)
105 Sustainable livestock production in the mountain agro-ecosystem of Nepal, 1992 (E)
106 Sustainable animal production from small farm systems in South-East Asia, 1993 (E)
107 Strategies for sustainable animal agriculture in developing countries, 1993 (E)
108 Evaluation of breeds and crosses of domestic animals, 1993 (E)
109 Bovine spongiform encephalopathy, 1993 (E)

Availability: March 1993

Ar	–	Arabic	Multil	–	Multilingual
C	–	Chinese	*		Out of print
E	–	English	**		In preparation
F	–	French			
P	–	Portuguese			
S	–	Spanish			

The FAO Technical Papers are available through the authorized FAO Sales Agents or directly from Distribution and Sales Section, FAO, Viale delle Terme di Caracalla, 00100 Rome, Italy.